Apple Resonance

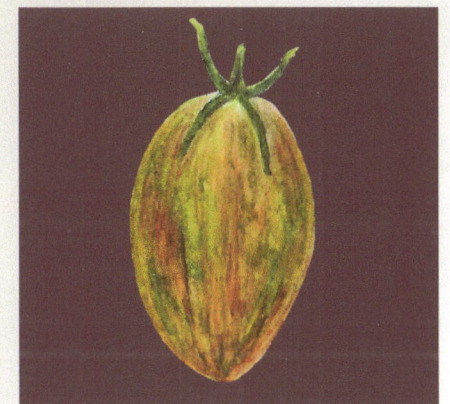 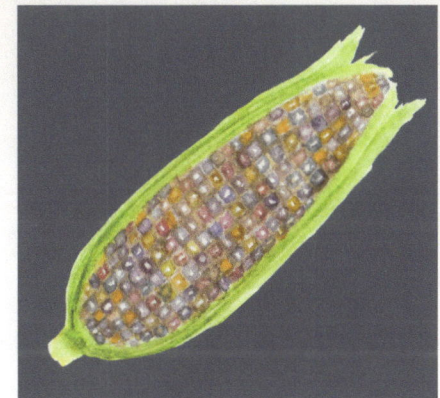 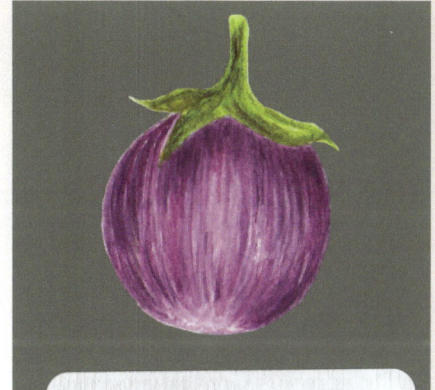

I Am SEED!

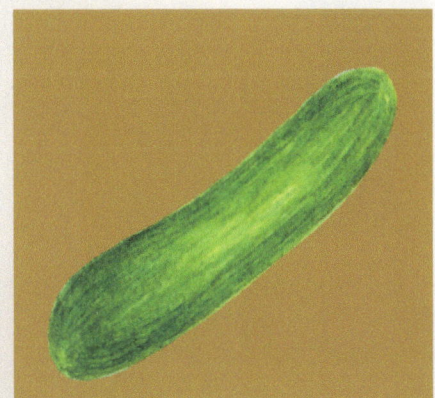 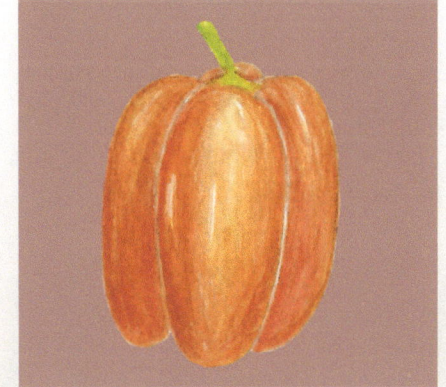 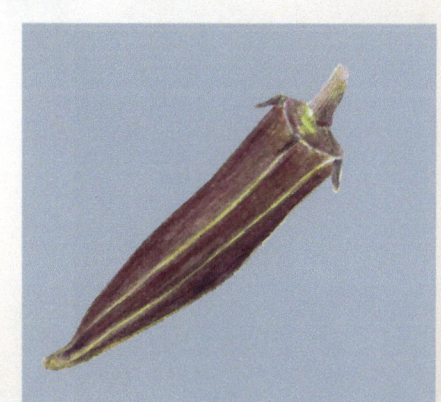

LemongrassPress.com

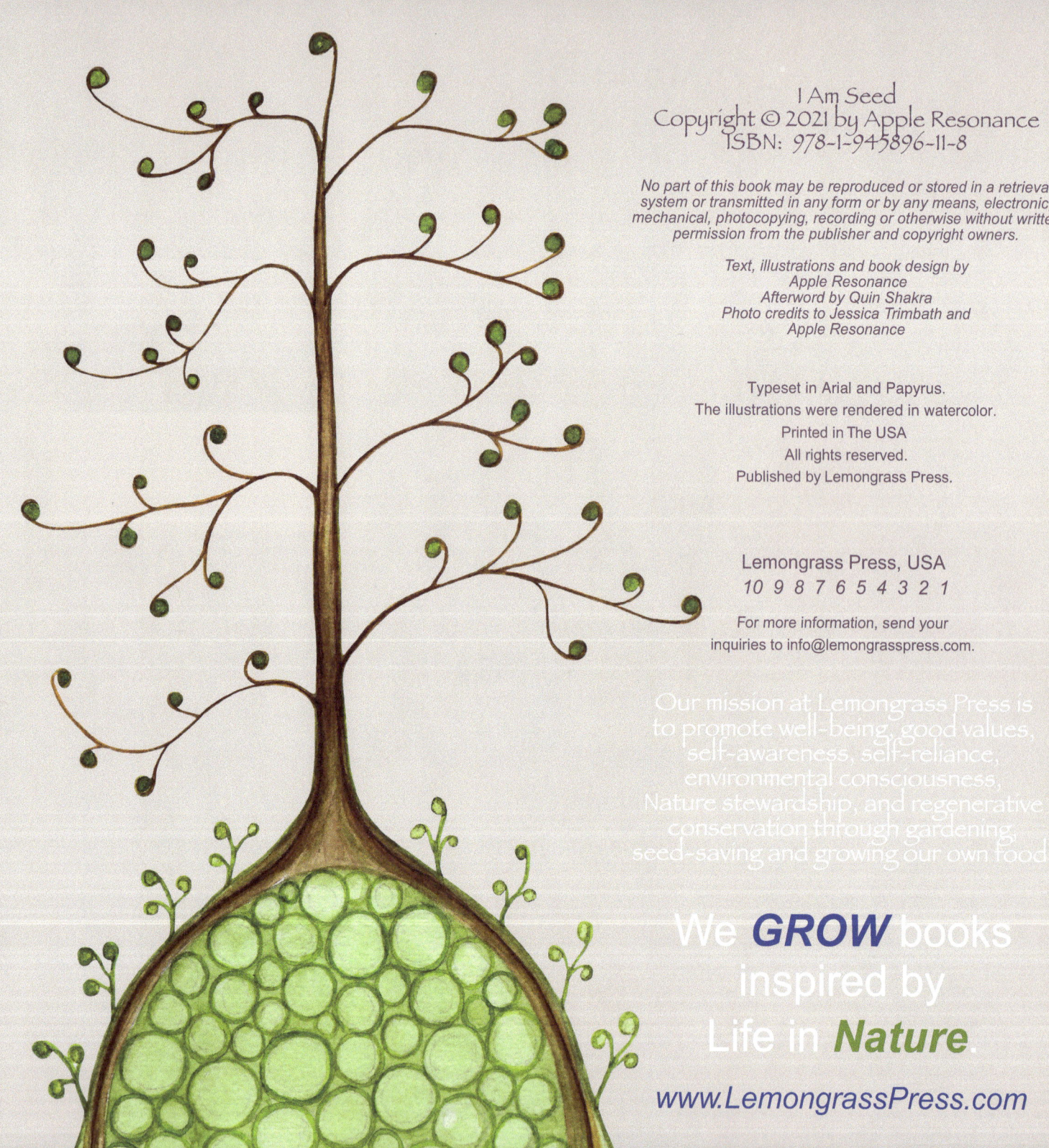

I Am Seed
Copyright © 2021 by Apple Resonance
ISBN: 978-1-945896-11-8

No part of this book may be reproduced or stored in a retrieval system or transmitted in any form or by any means, electronic, mechanical, photocopying, recording or otherwise without written permission from the publisher and copyright owners.

Text, illustrations and book design by
Apple Resonance
Afterword by Quin Shakra
Photo credits to Jessica Trimbath and
Apple Resonance

Typeset in Arial and Papyrus.
The illustrations were rendered in watercolor.
Printed in The USA
All rights reserved.
Published by Lemongrass Press.

Lemongrass Press, USA
10 9 8 7 6 5 4 3 2 1

For more information, send your
inquiries to info@lemongrasspress.com

Our mission at Lemongrass Press is to promote well-being, good values, self-awareness, self-reliance, environmental consciousness, Nature stewardship, and regenerative conservation through gardening, seed-saving and growing our own food.

We **GROW** books
inspired by
Life in *Nature*.

www.LemongrassPress.com

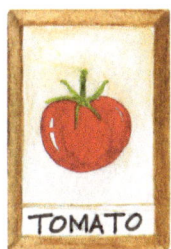

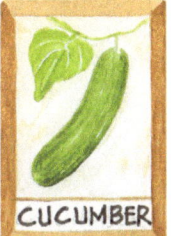
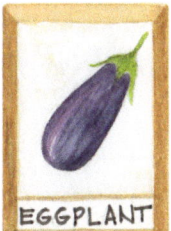
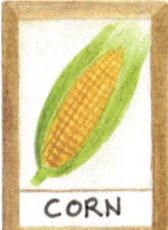
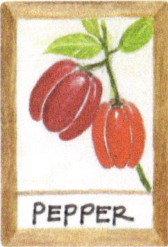

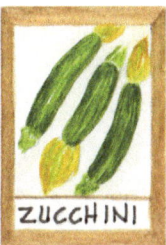
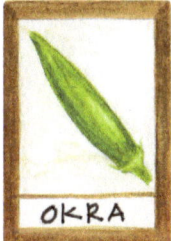
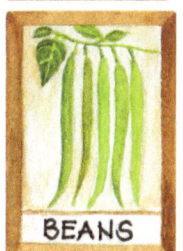

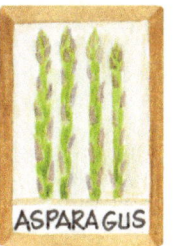
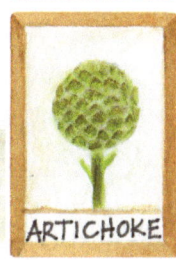

To my dearest fruits...
Michael Anthony and Anastasya Mikaela.

To all the SEED LOVERS.
To all the SEED-SAVERS.
To all the SEED-KEEPERS.
To all the SEED STEWARDS.

The CO-CREATORS of the EARTH.
Mother Nature loves YOU.

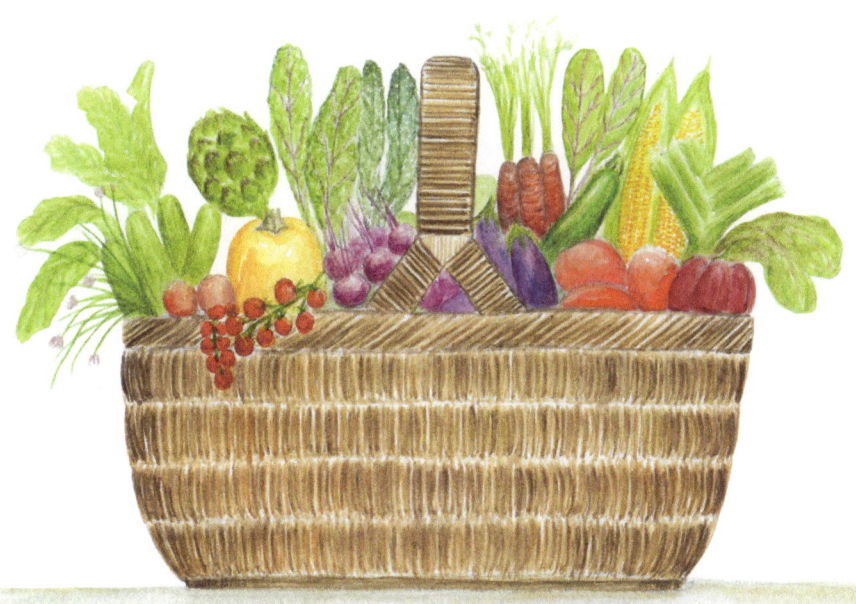

Save Seeds, Save the Future.

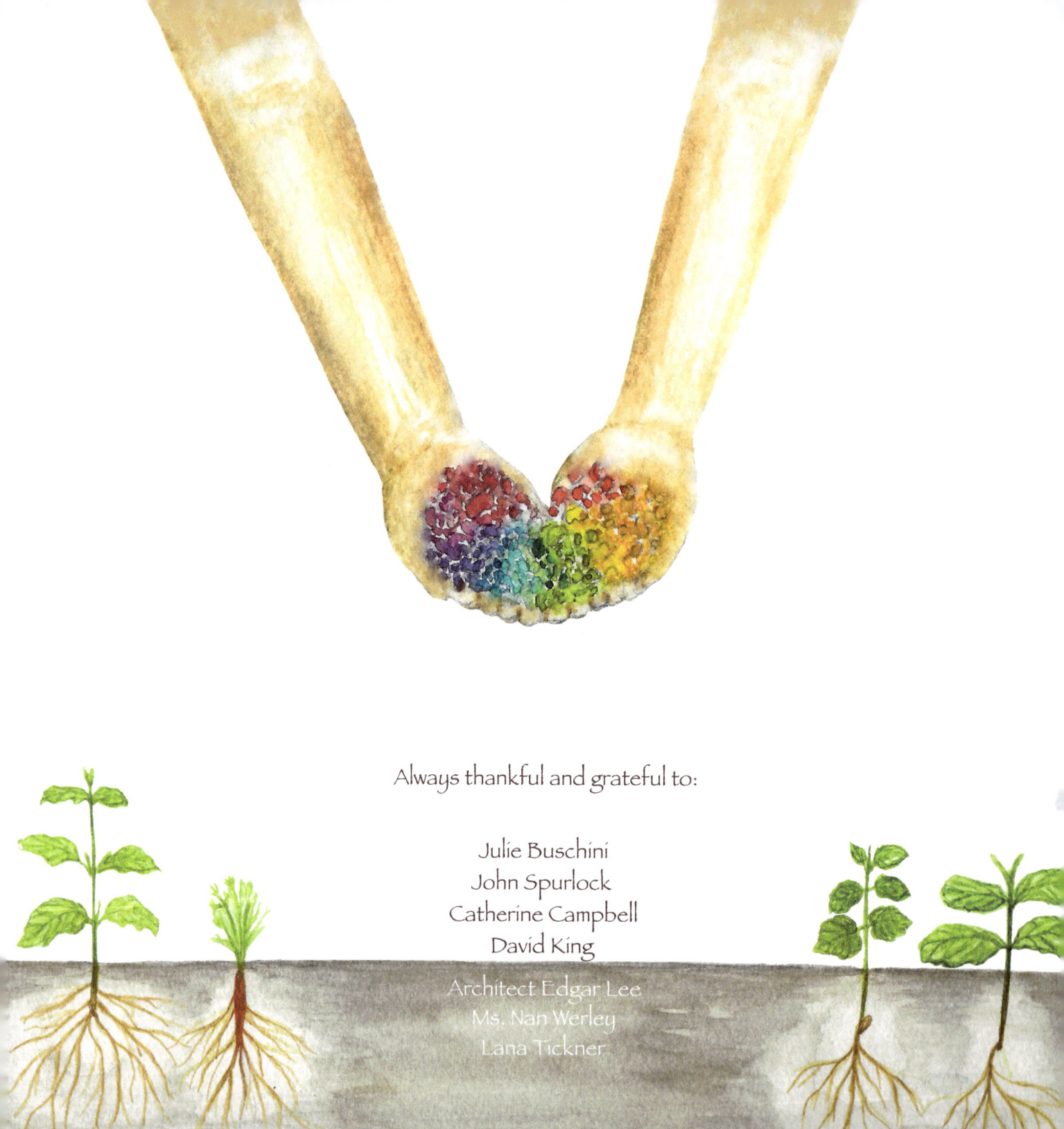

Always thankful and grateful to:

Julie Buschini
John Spurlock
Catherine Campbell
David King

Architect Edgar Lee
Ms. Nan Werley
Lana Tickner

Sow yourself in GOOD SOIL,
dear GOOD SEED.
Let the GARDEN within YOU,
GROW what you may need!

— Apple Resonance
"I Am Quinoa!",
Earth Day 2020

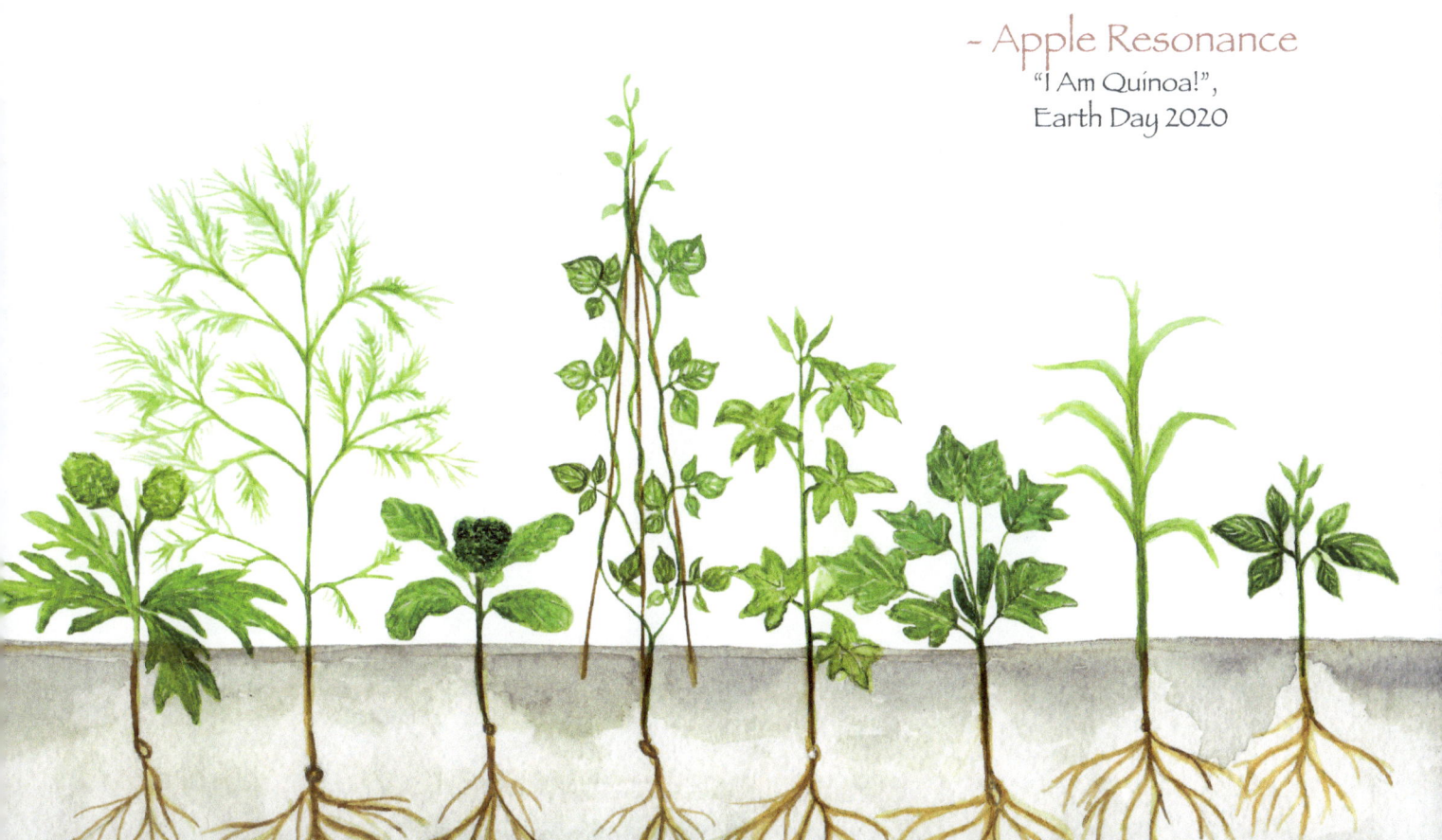

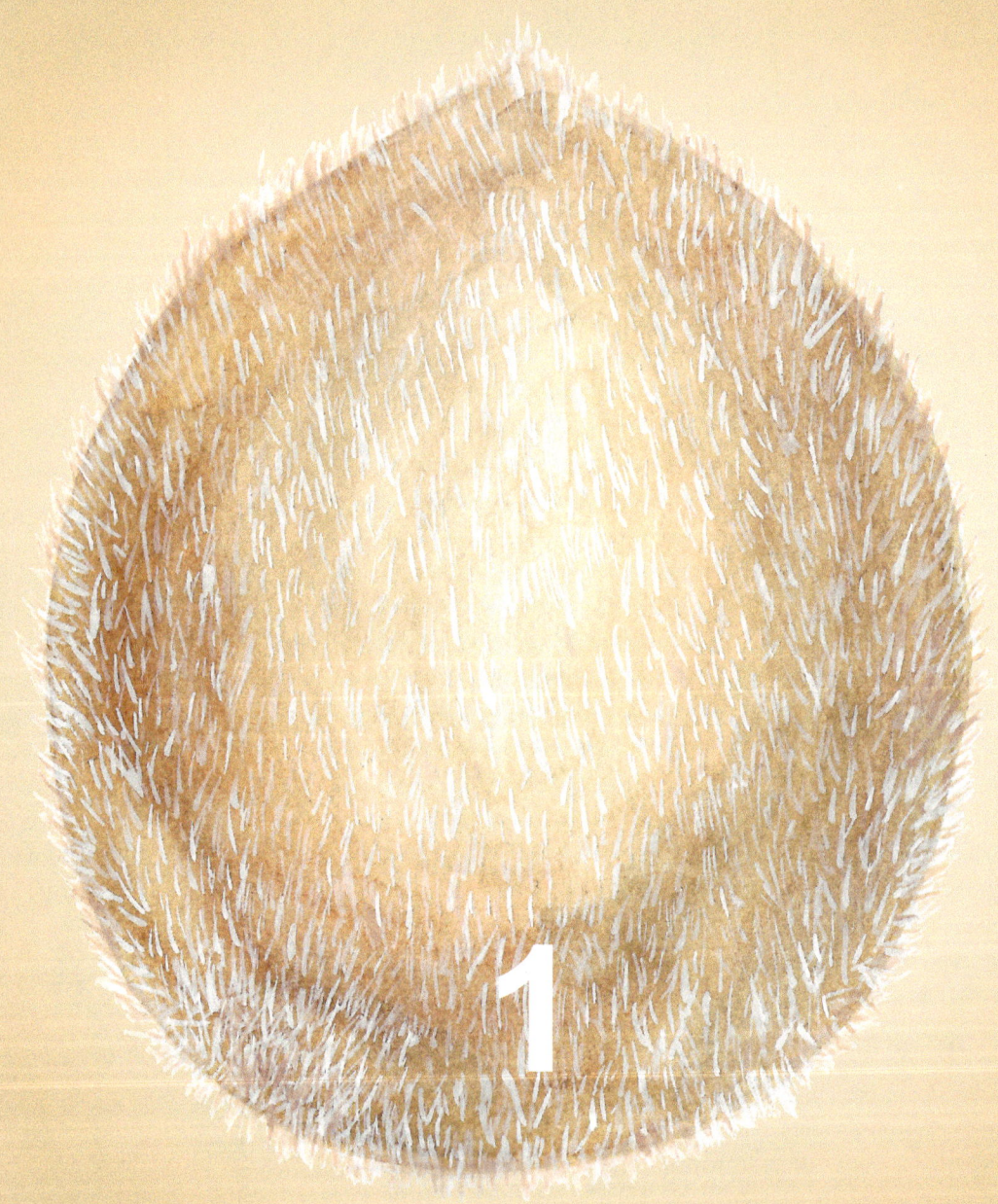

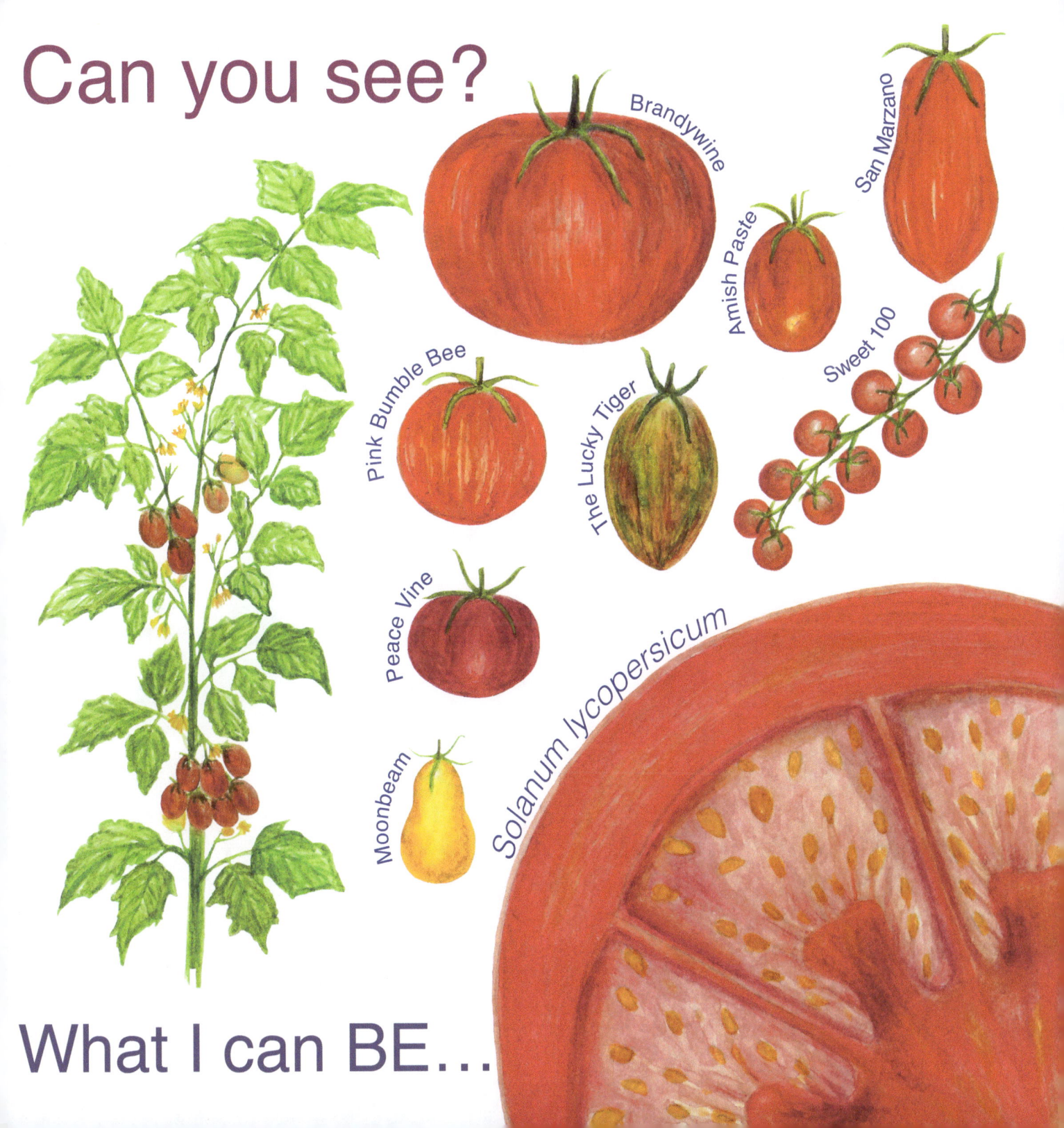

I am a *SEED*.

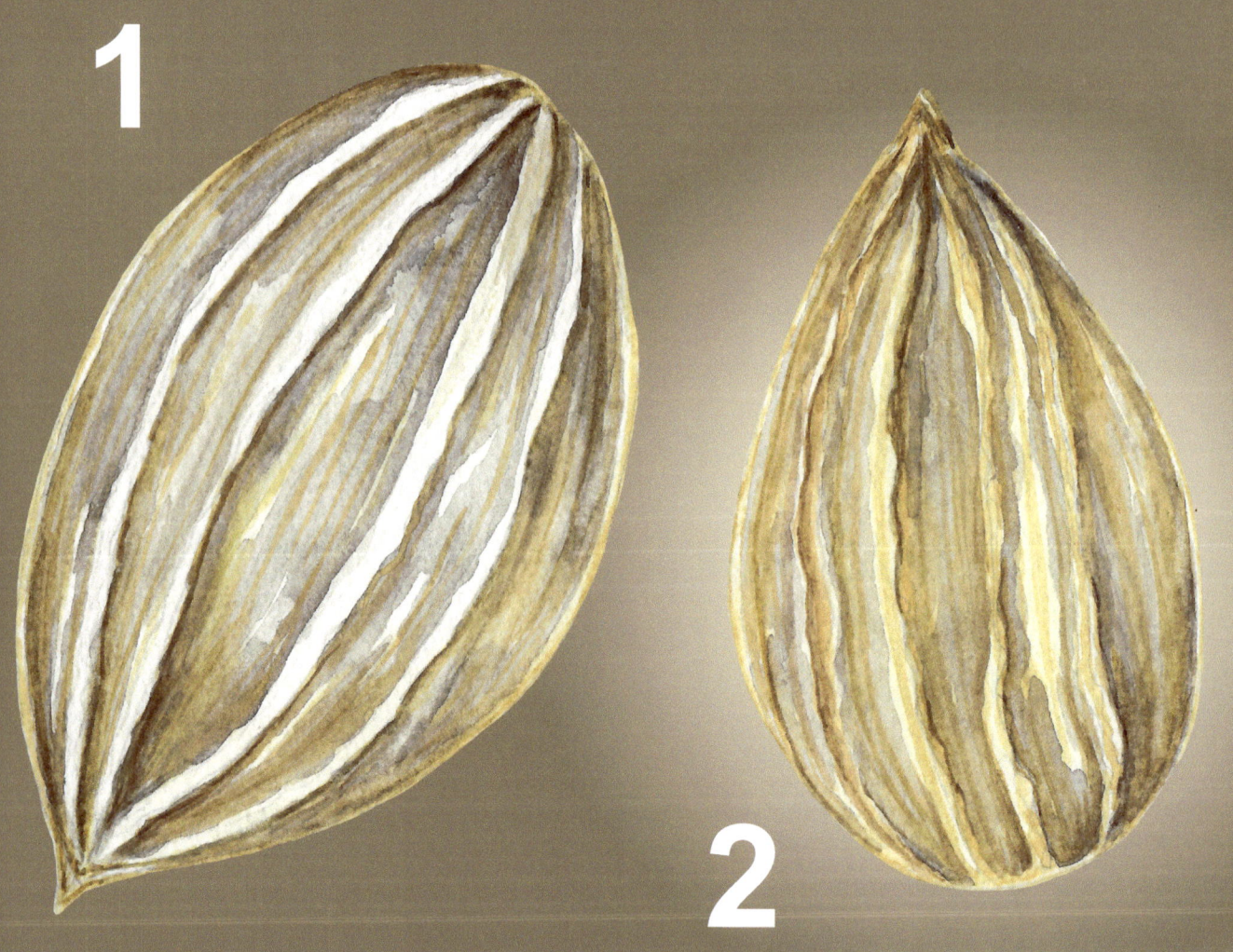

...a *CARROT* seed.

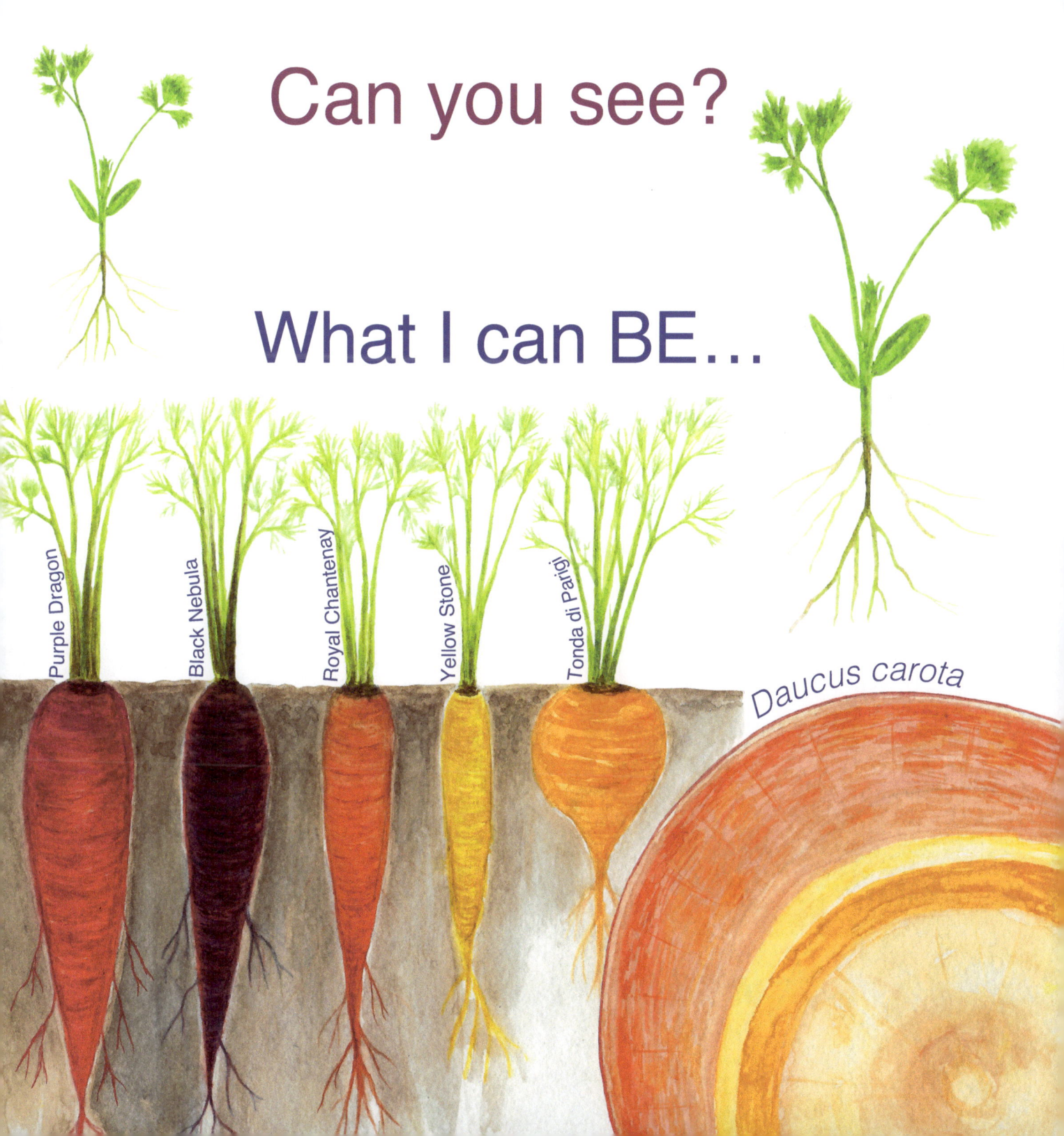

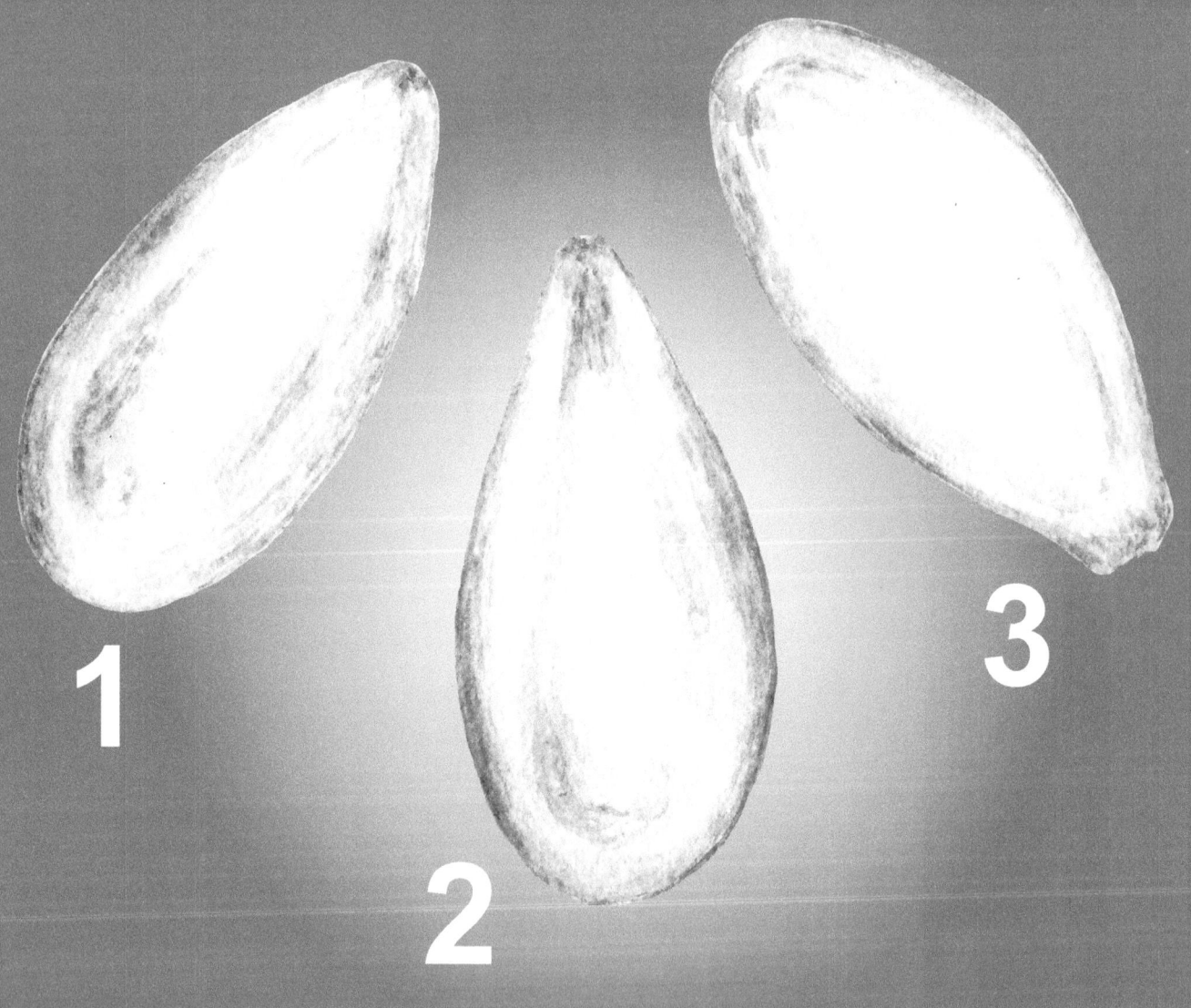

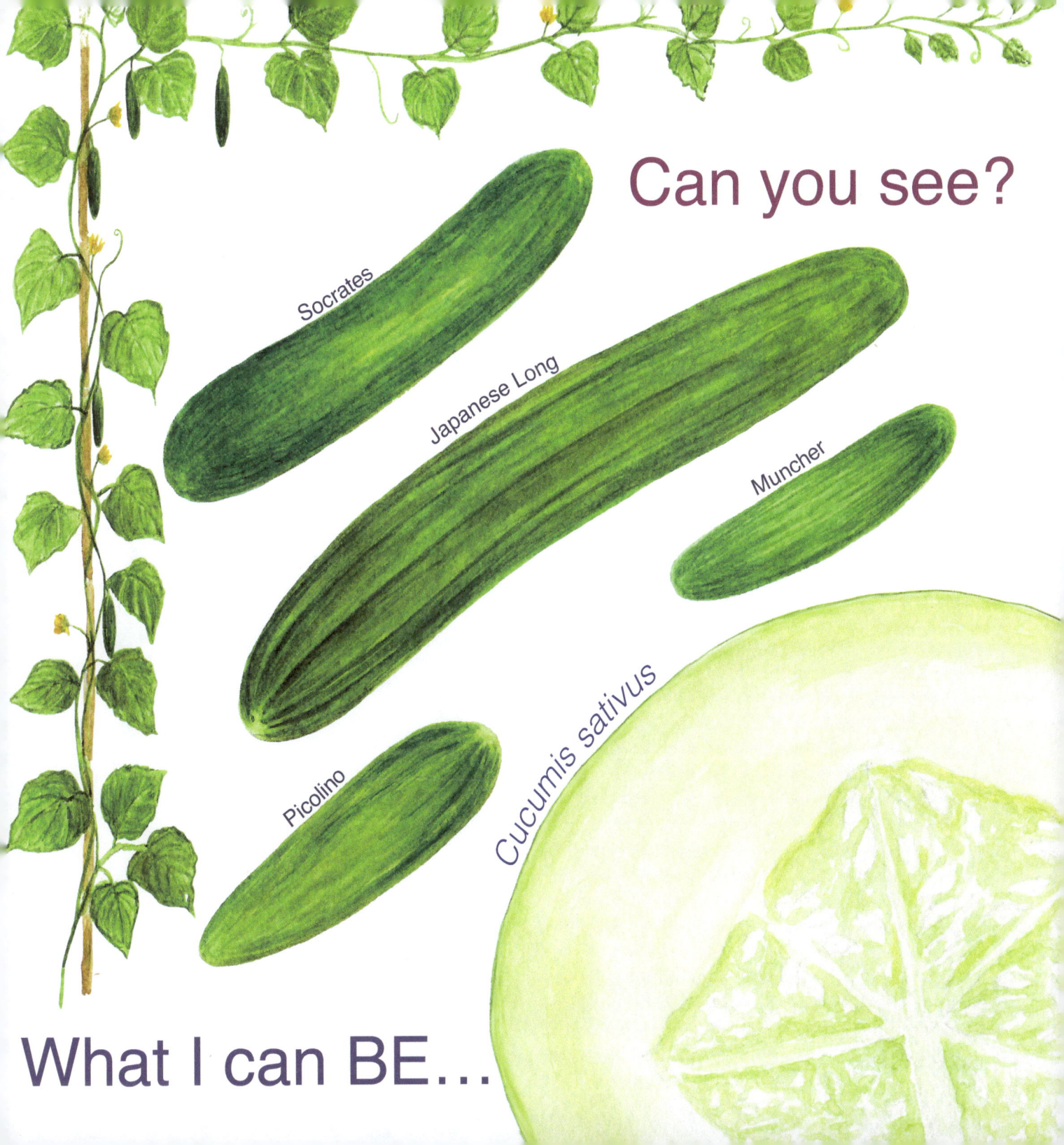

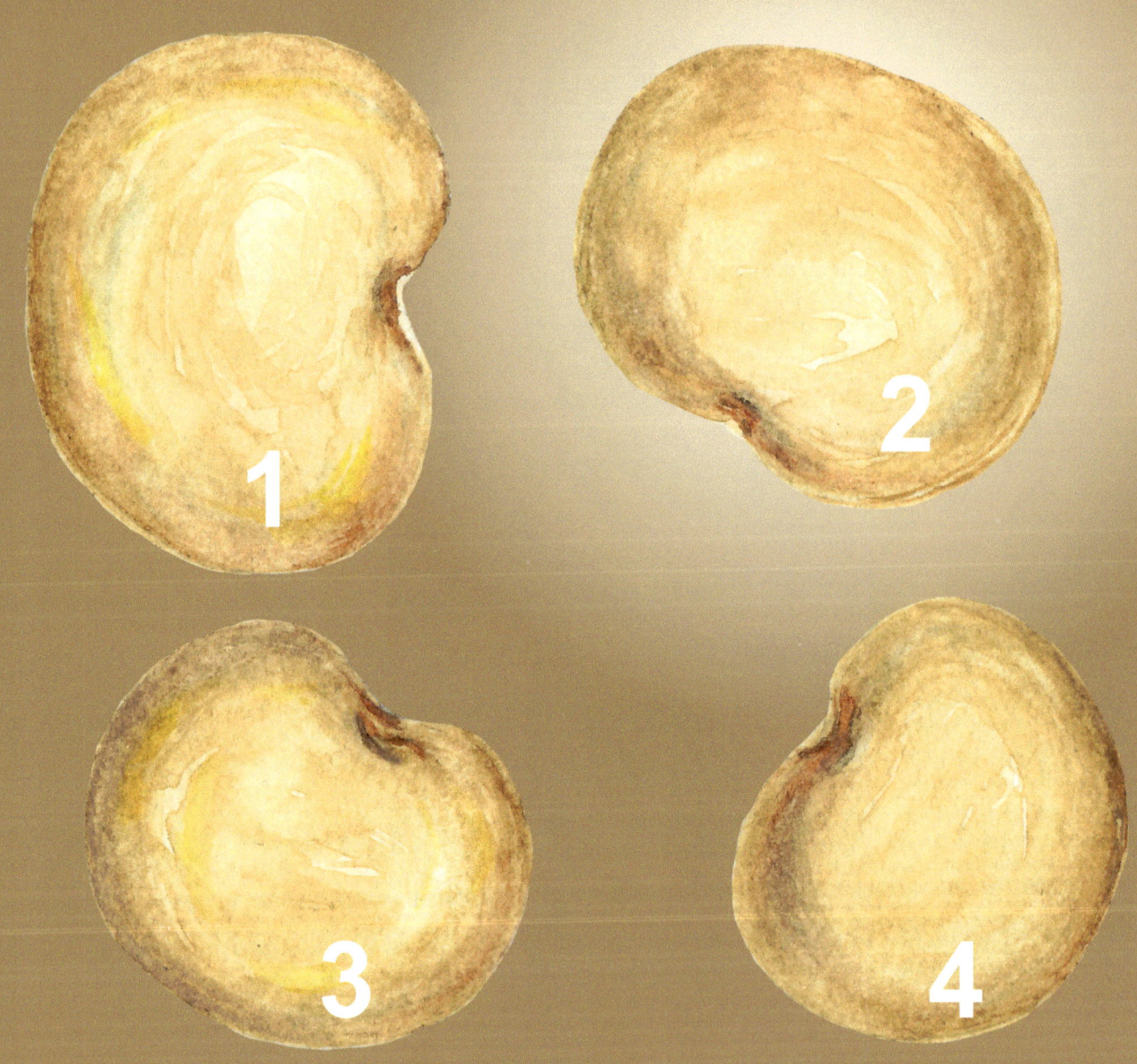

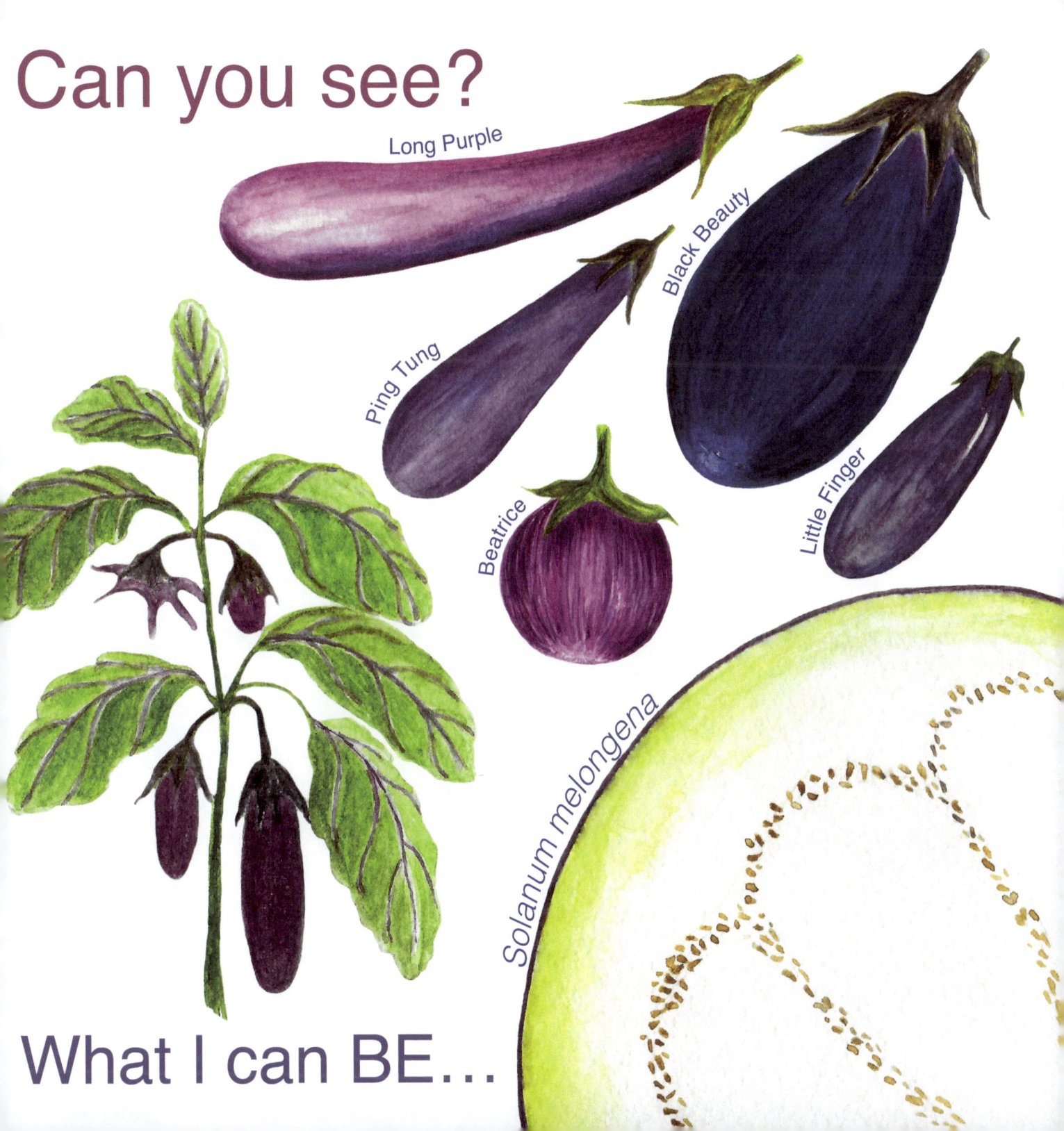

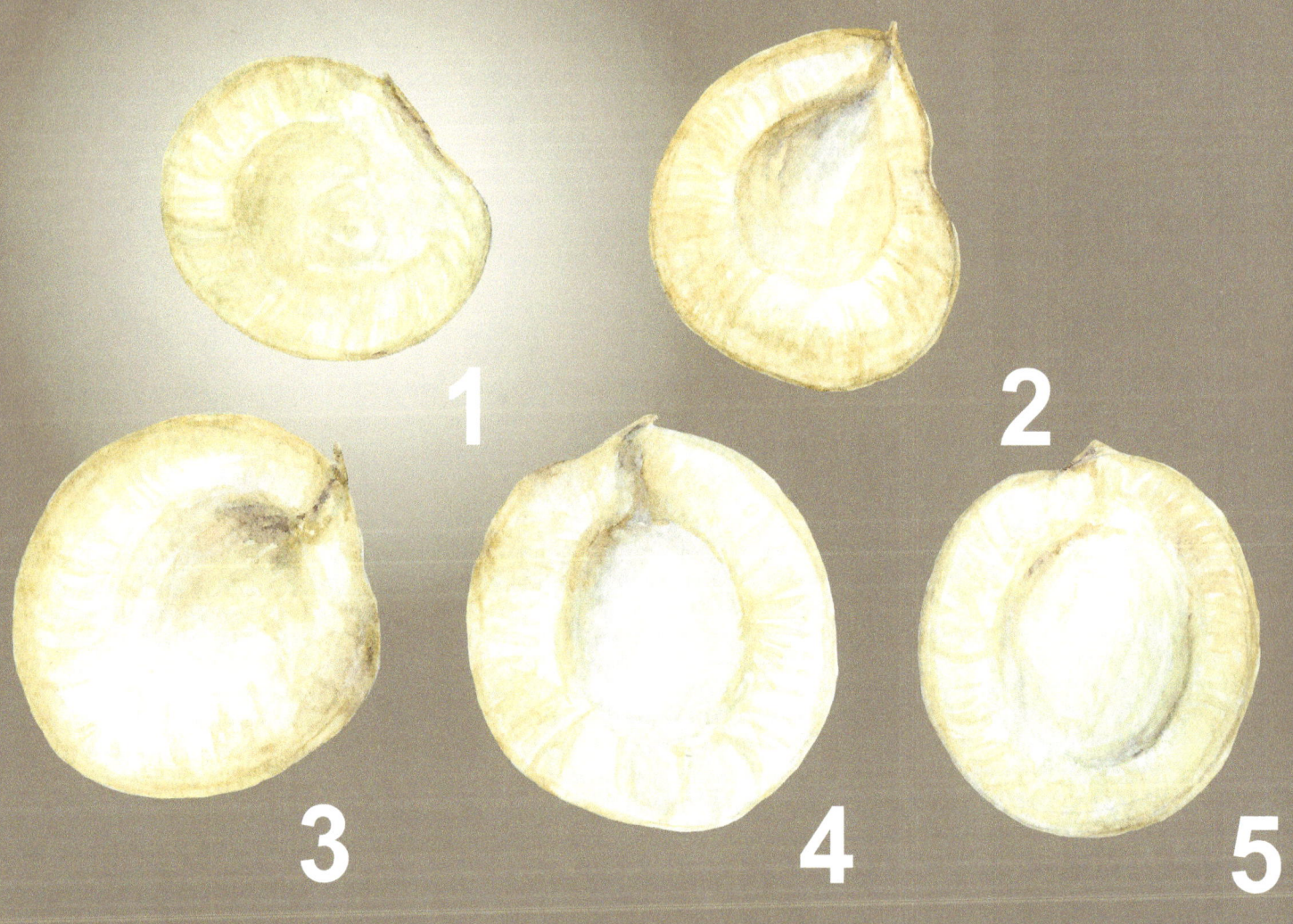

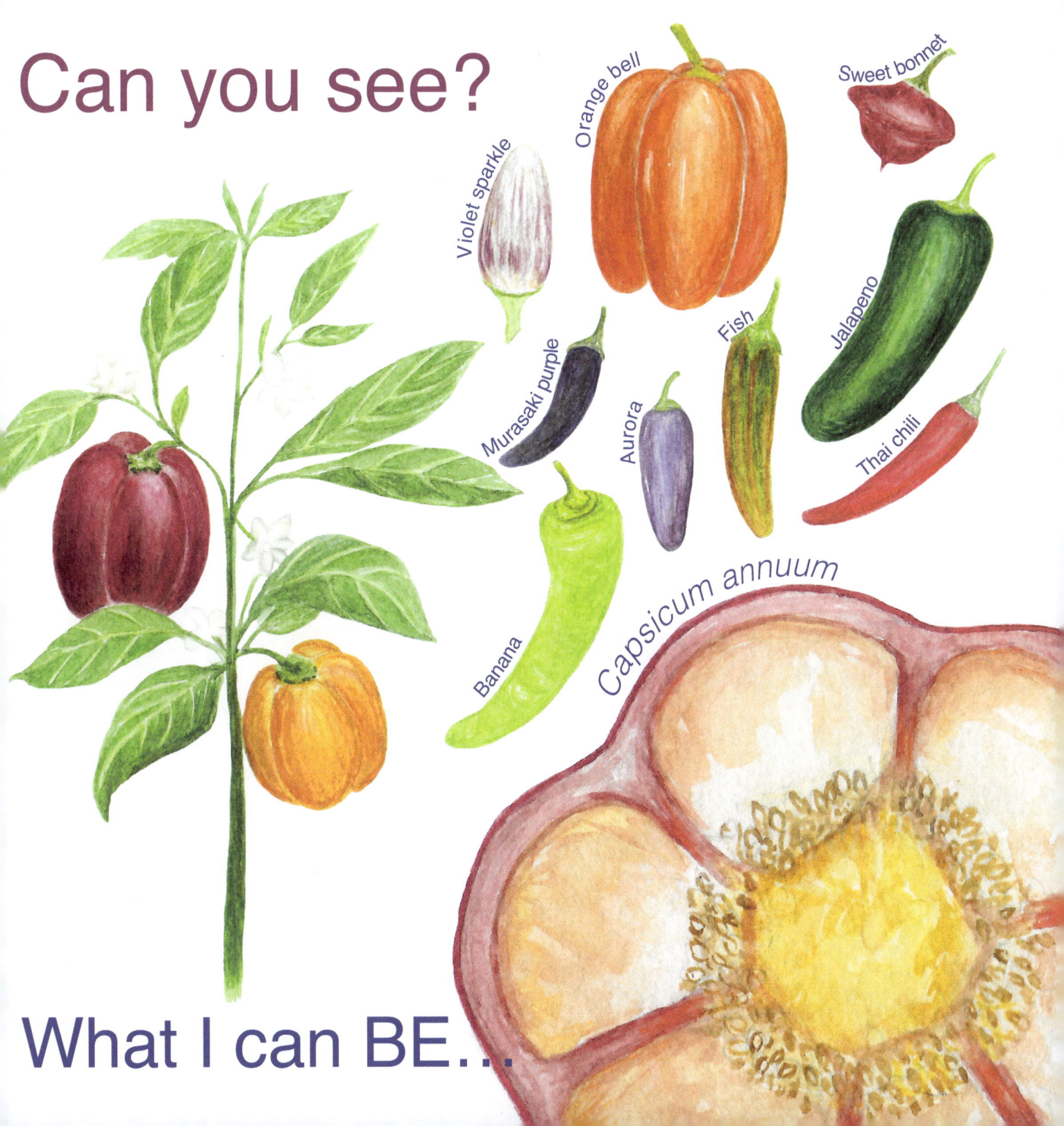

I am a *SEED*.

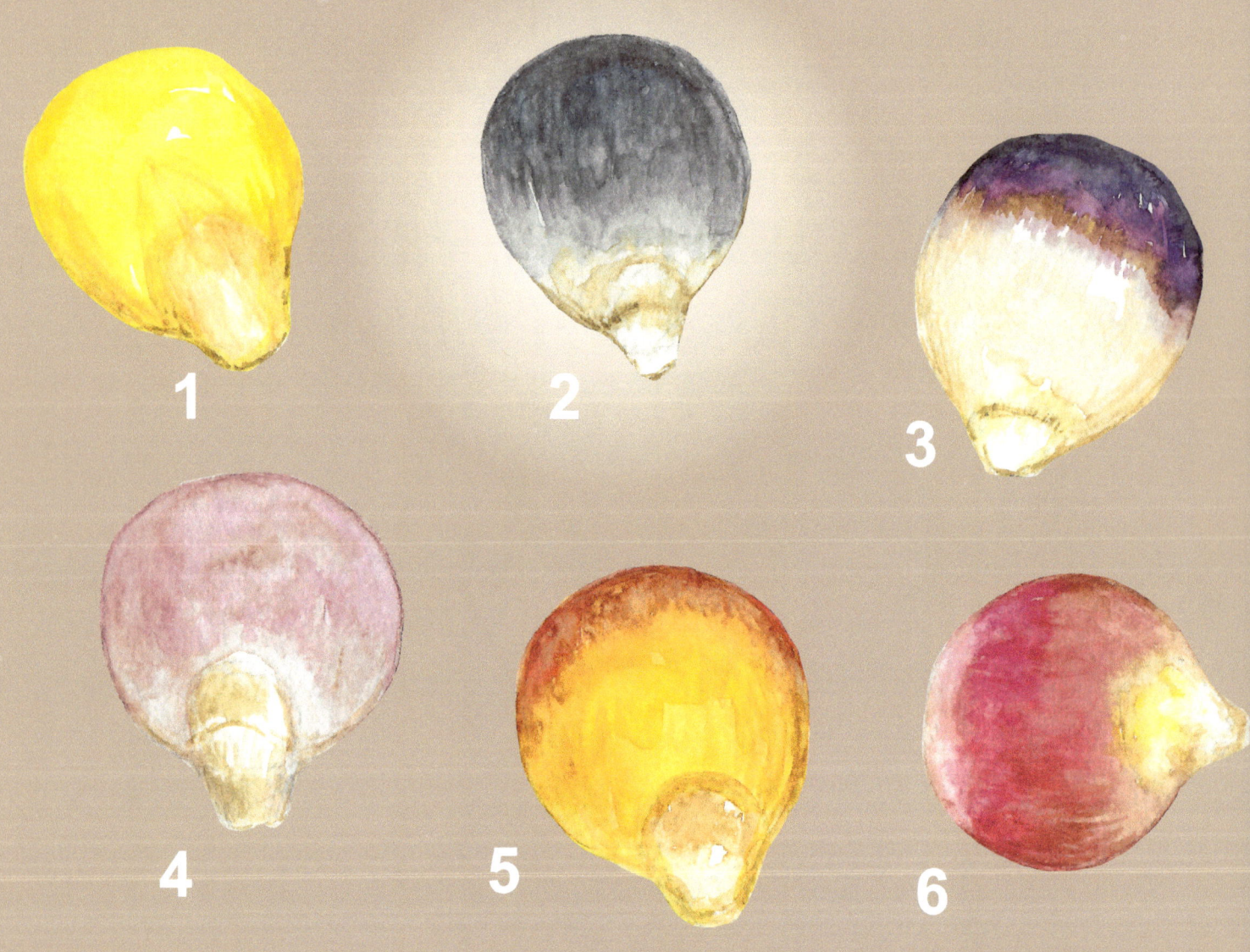

...a *CORN* seed.

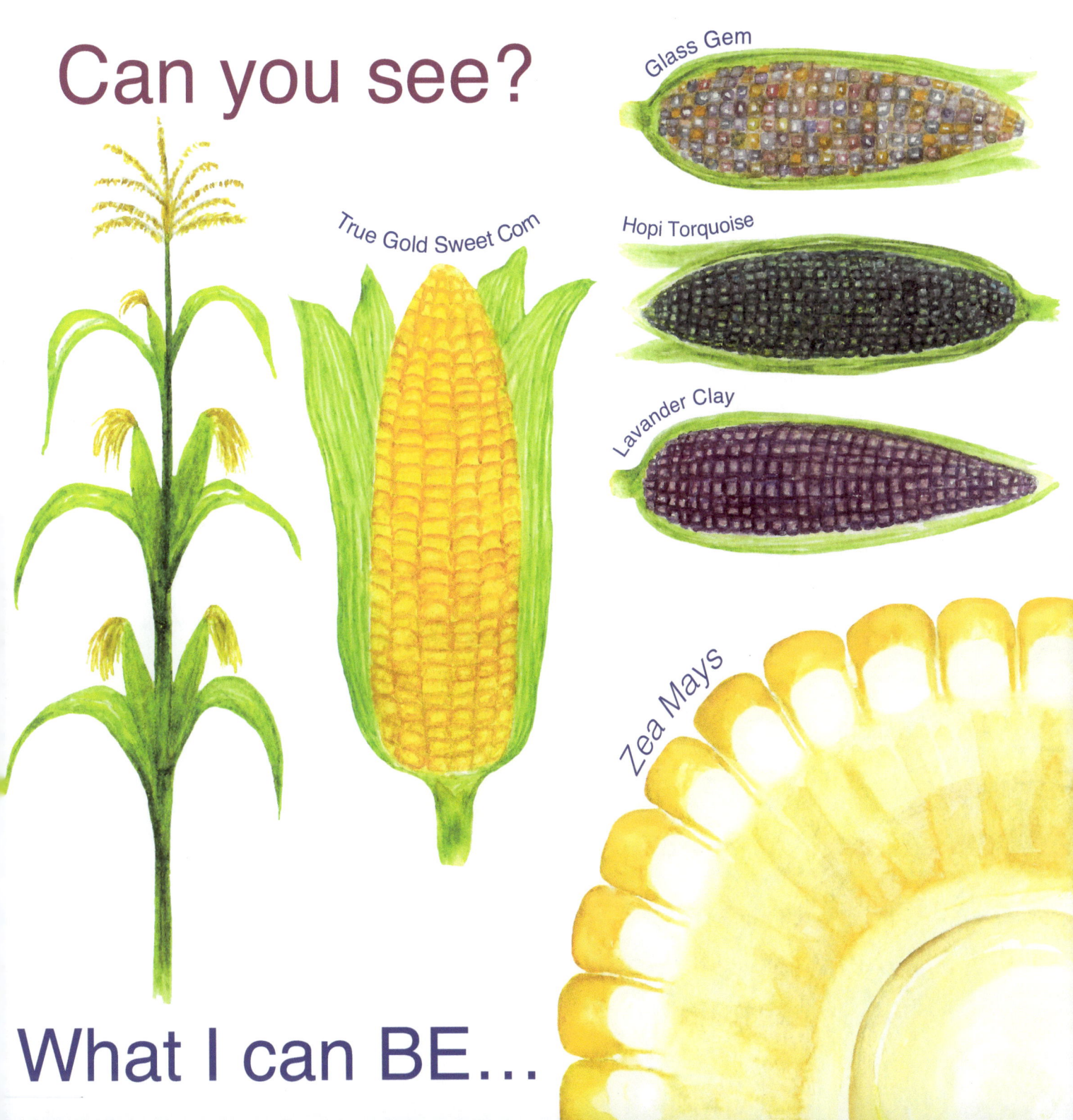

I am a SEED.

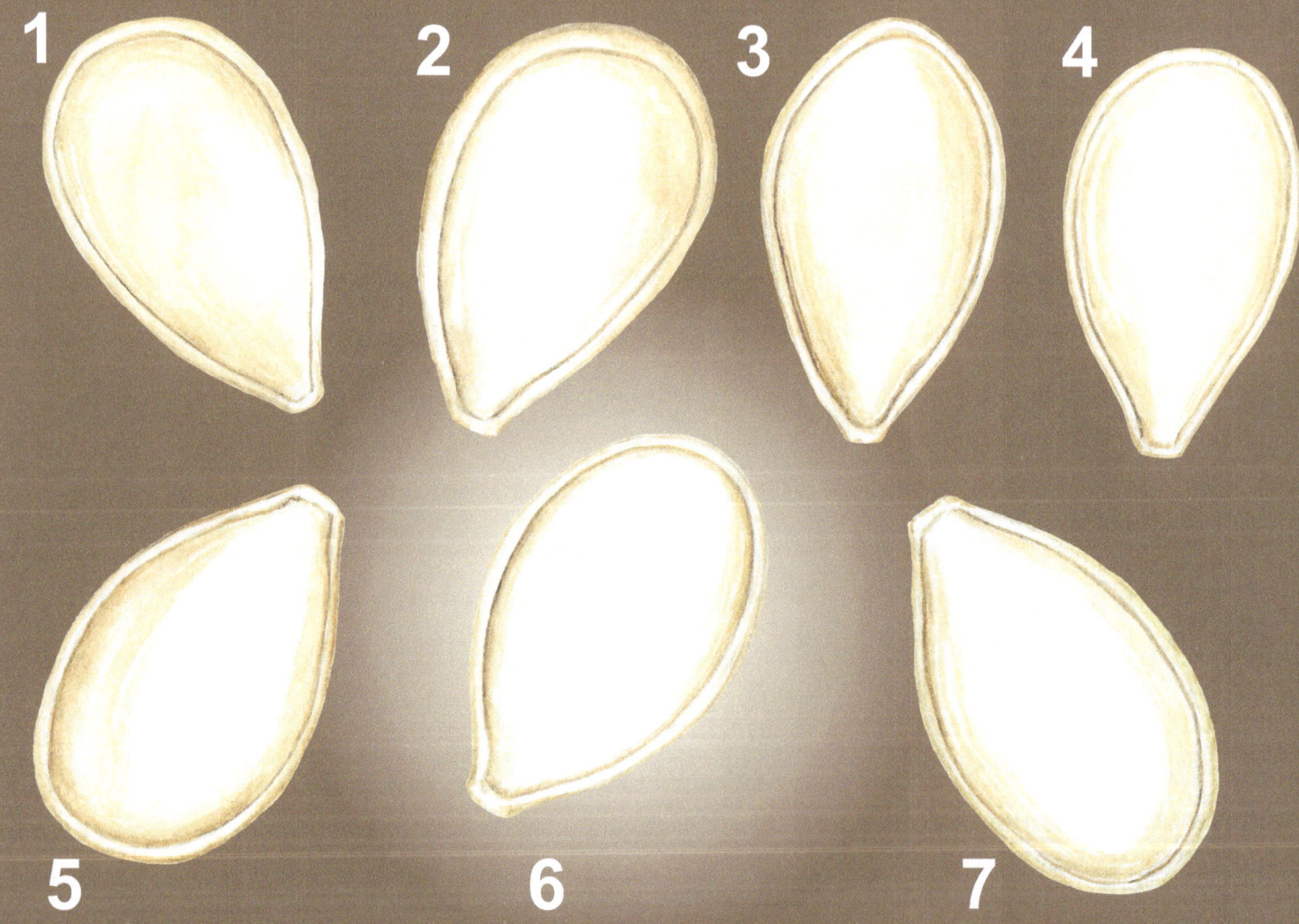

...a ZUCCHINI seed.

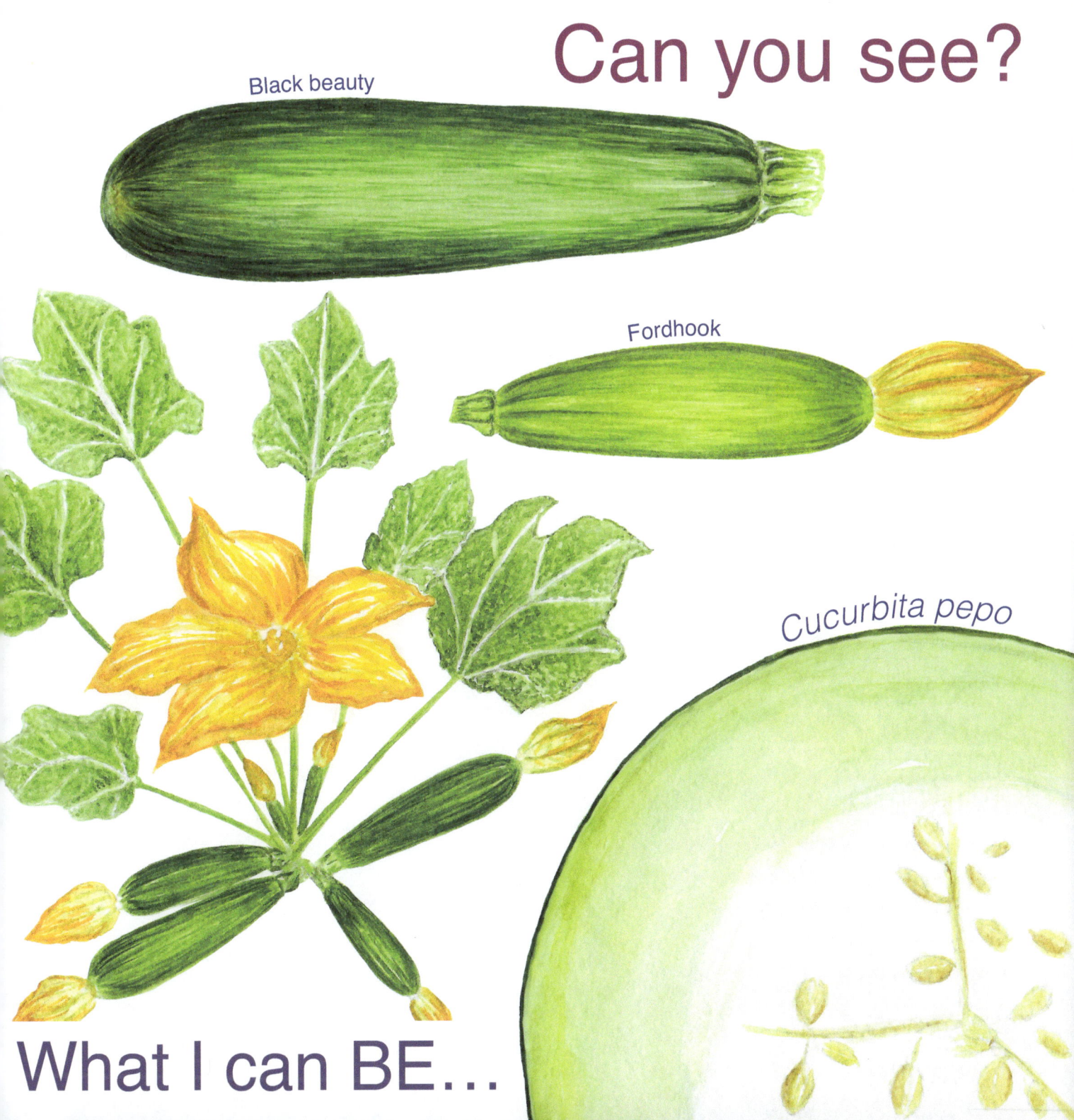

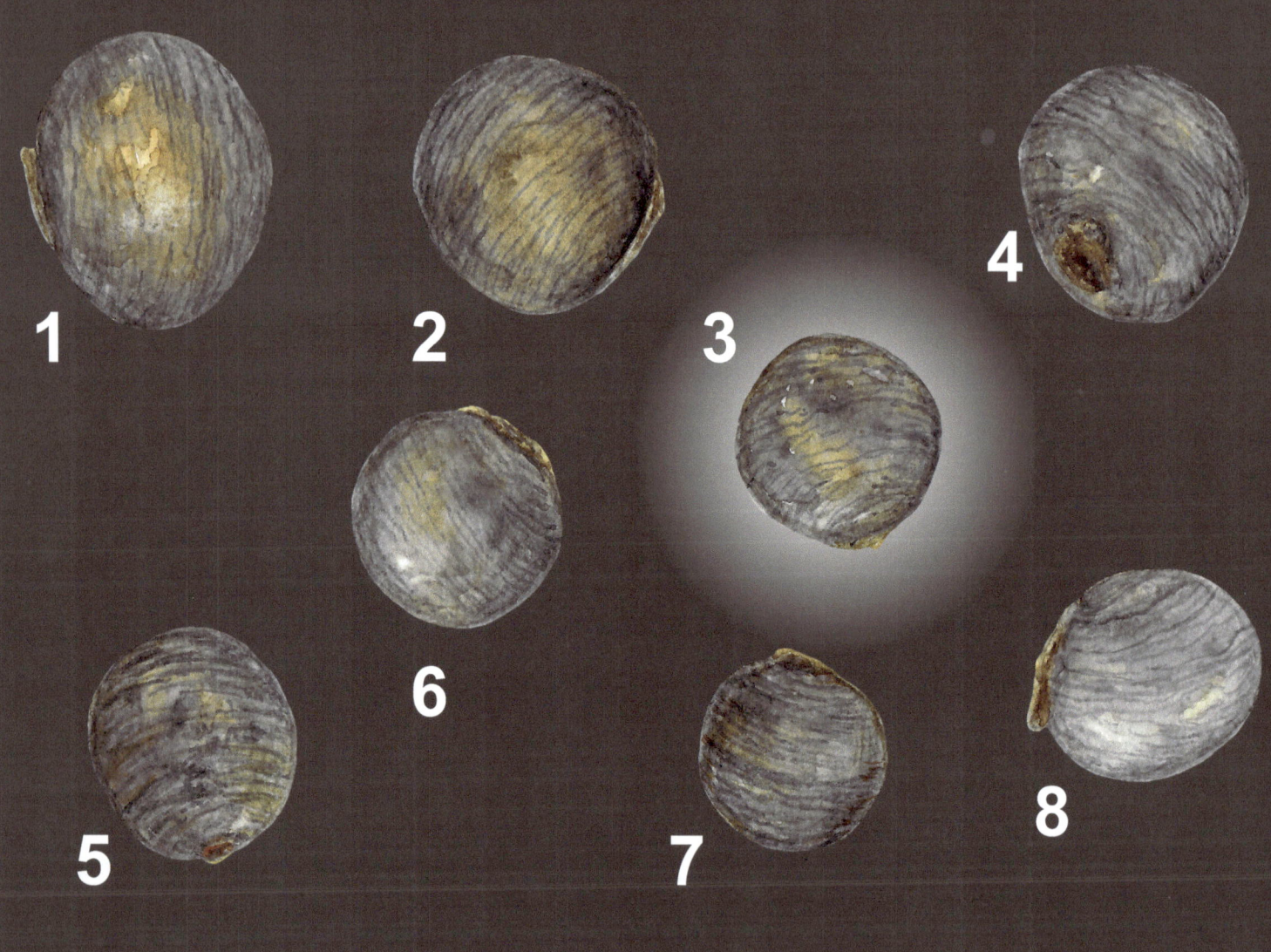

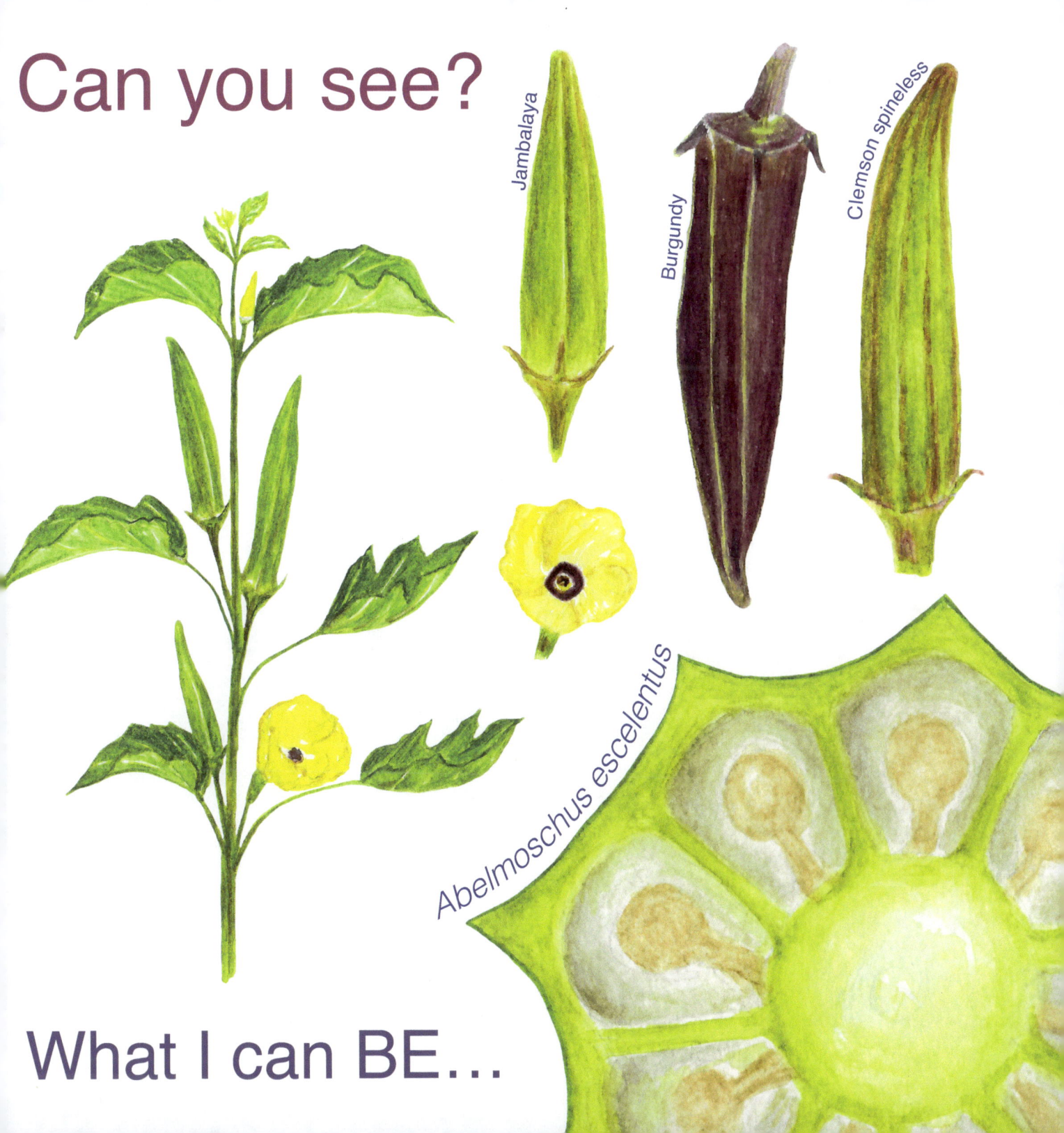

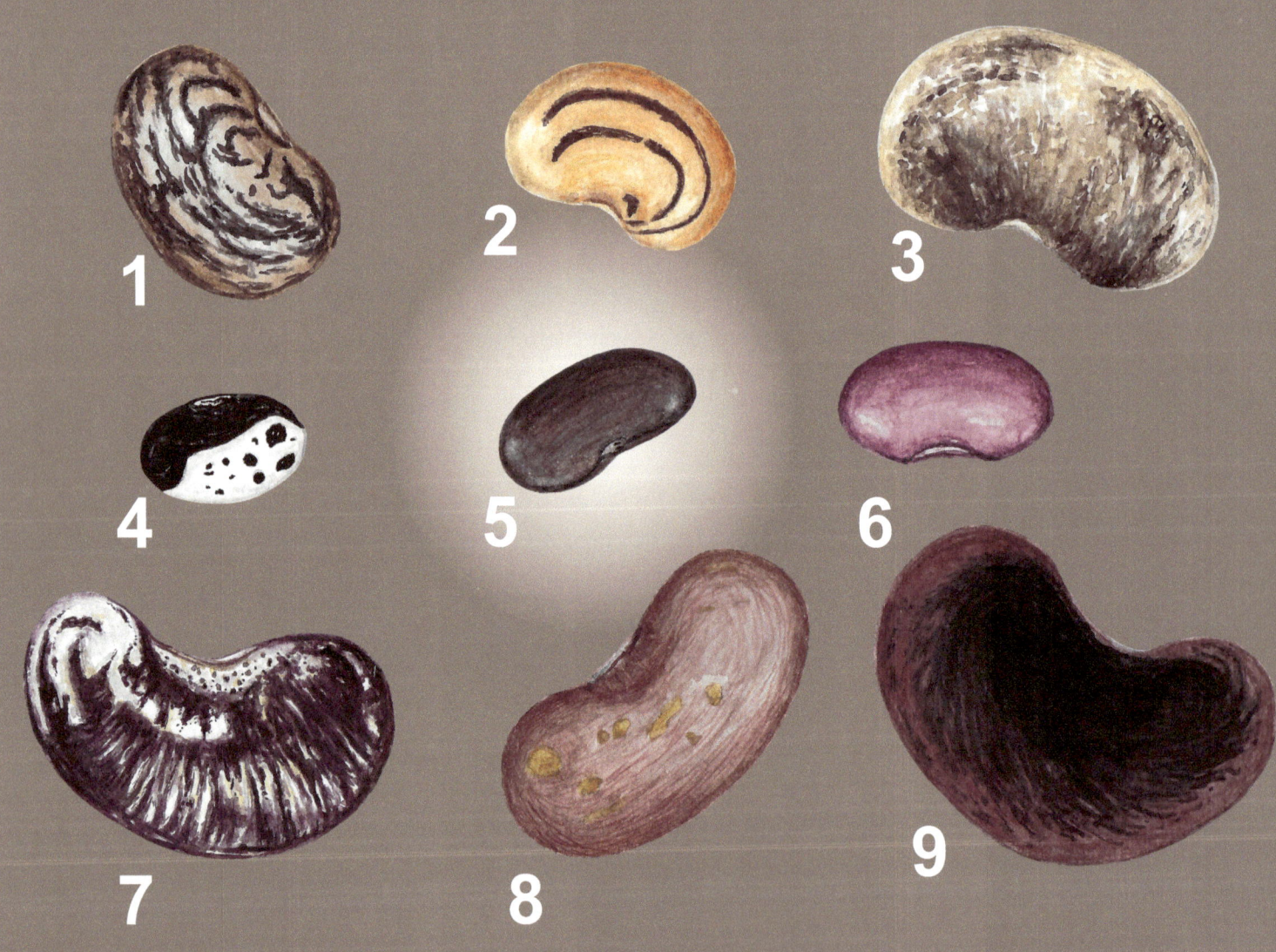

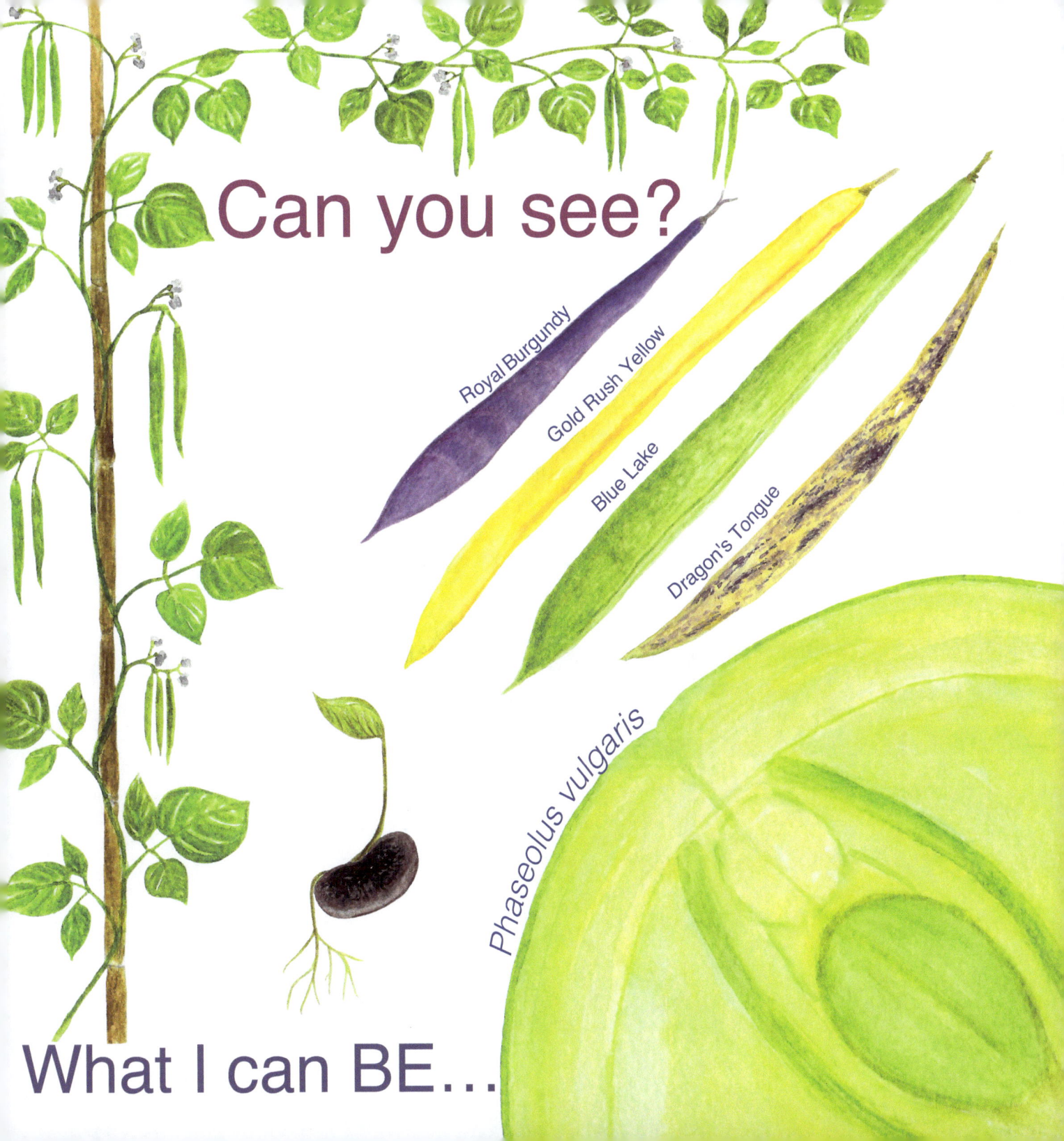

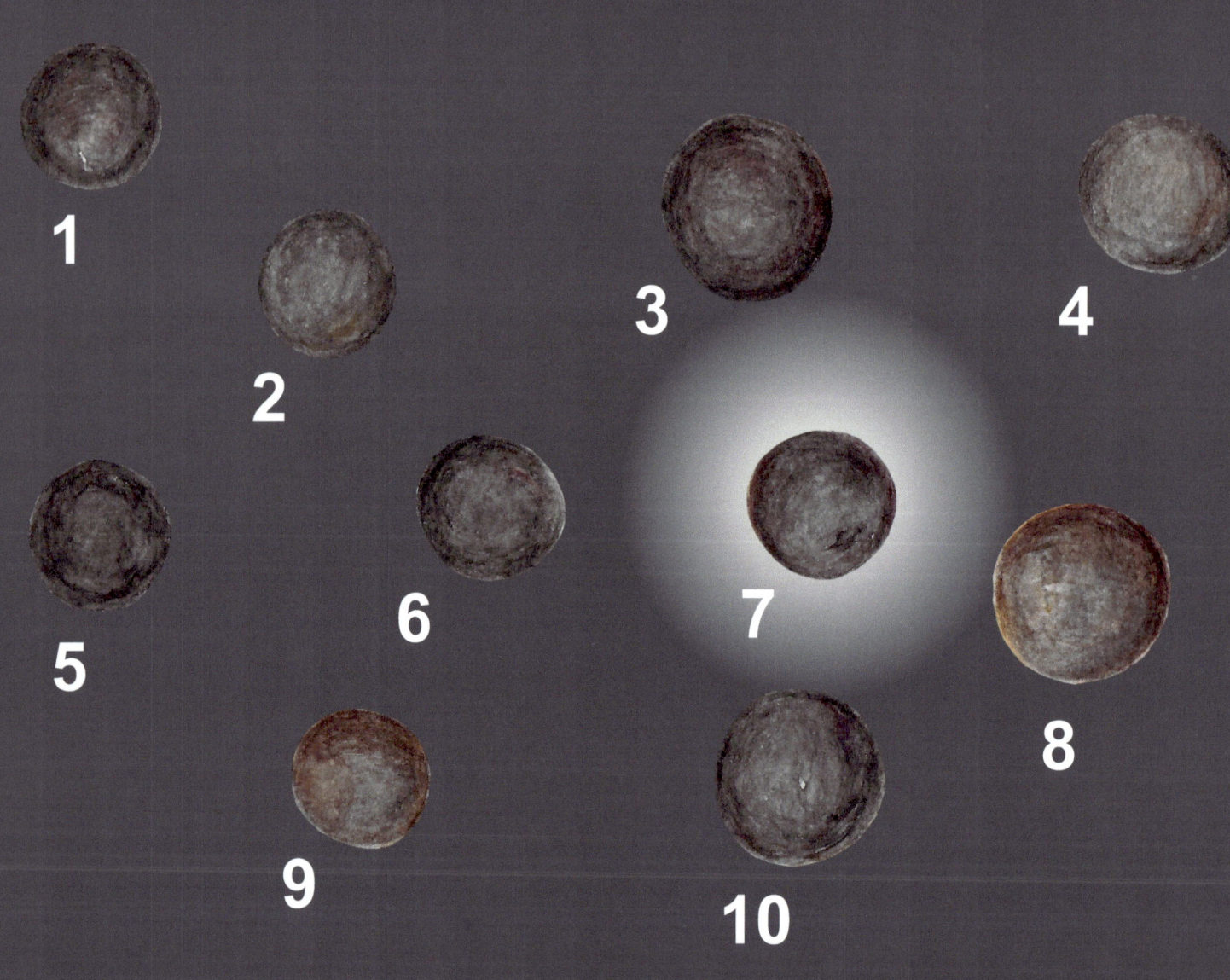

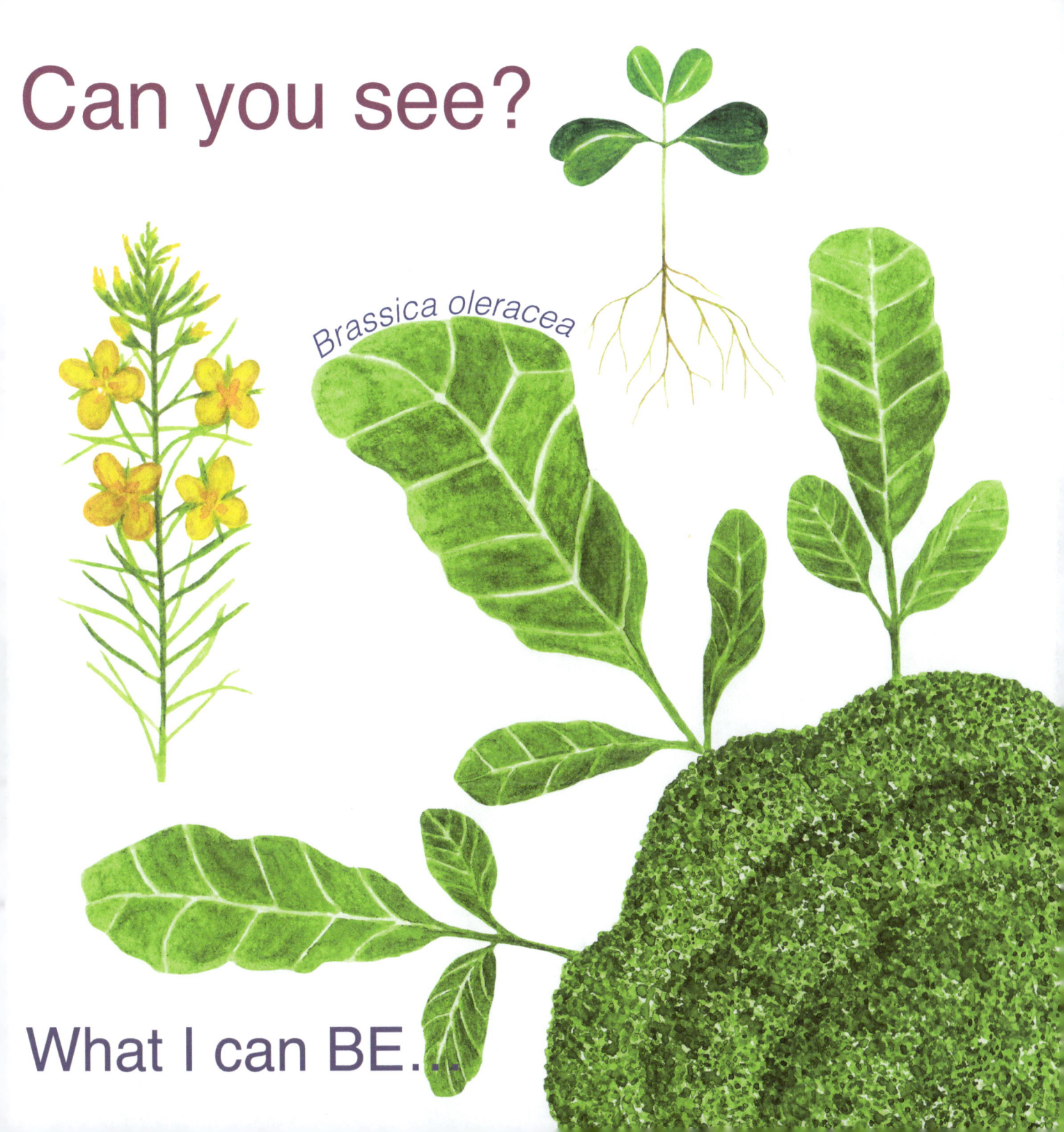

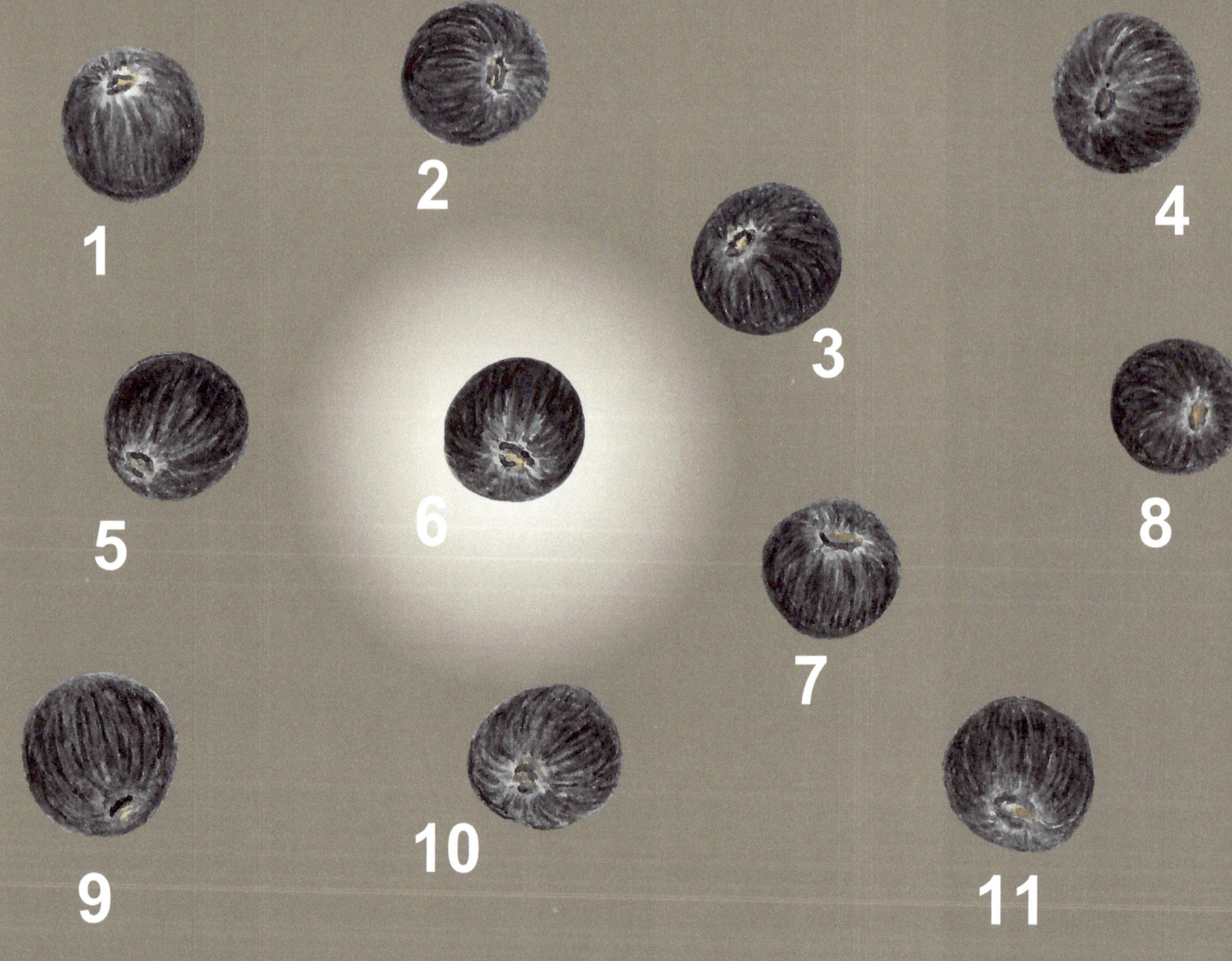

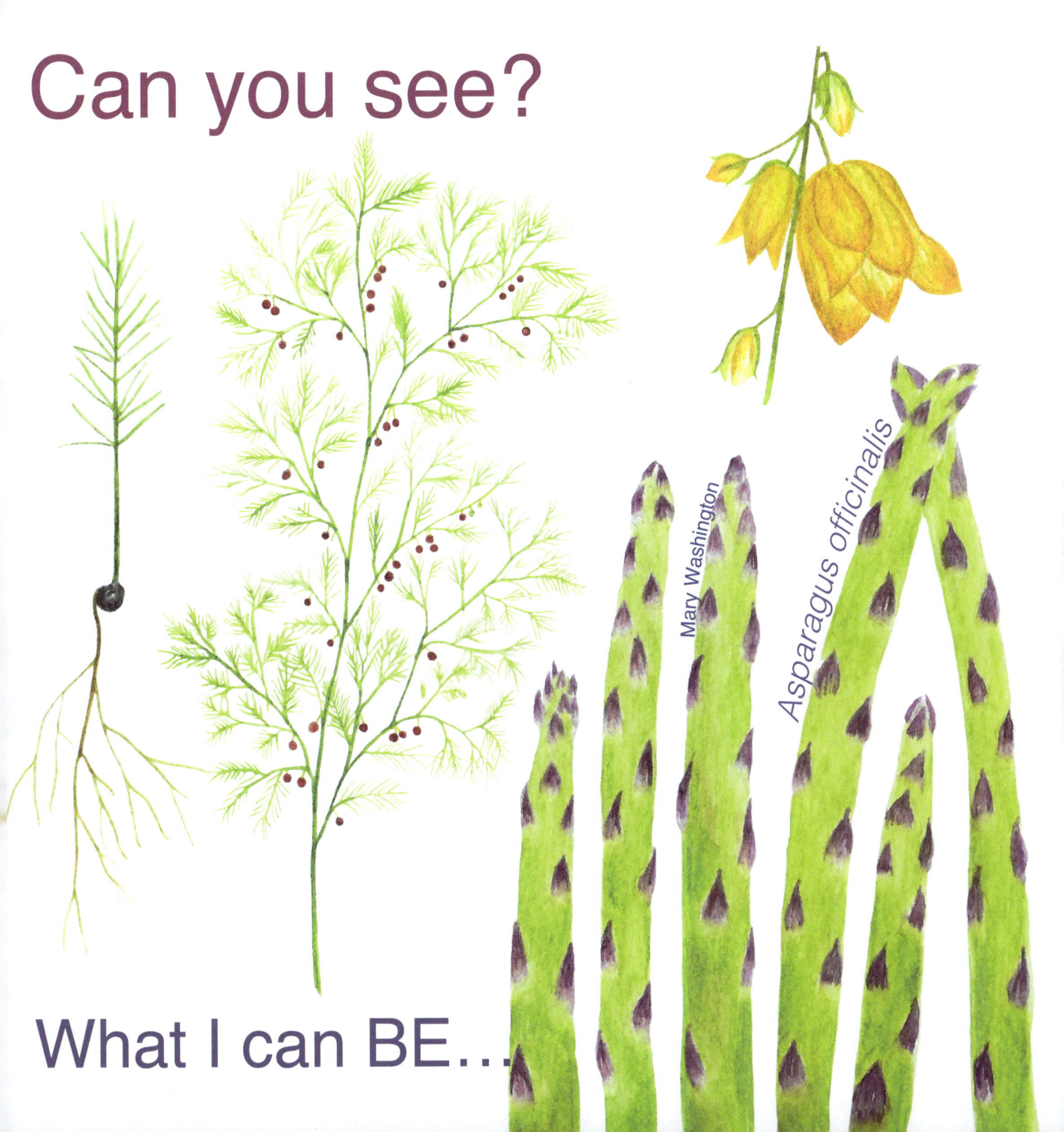

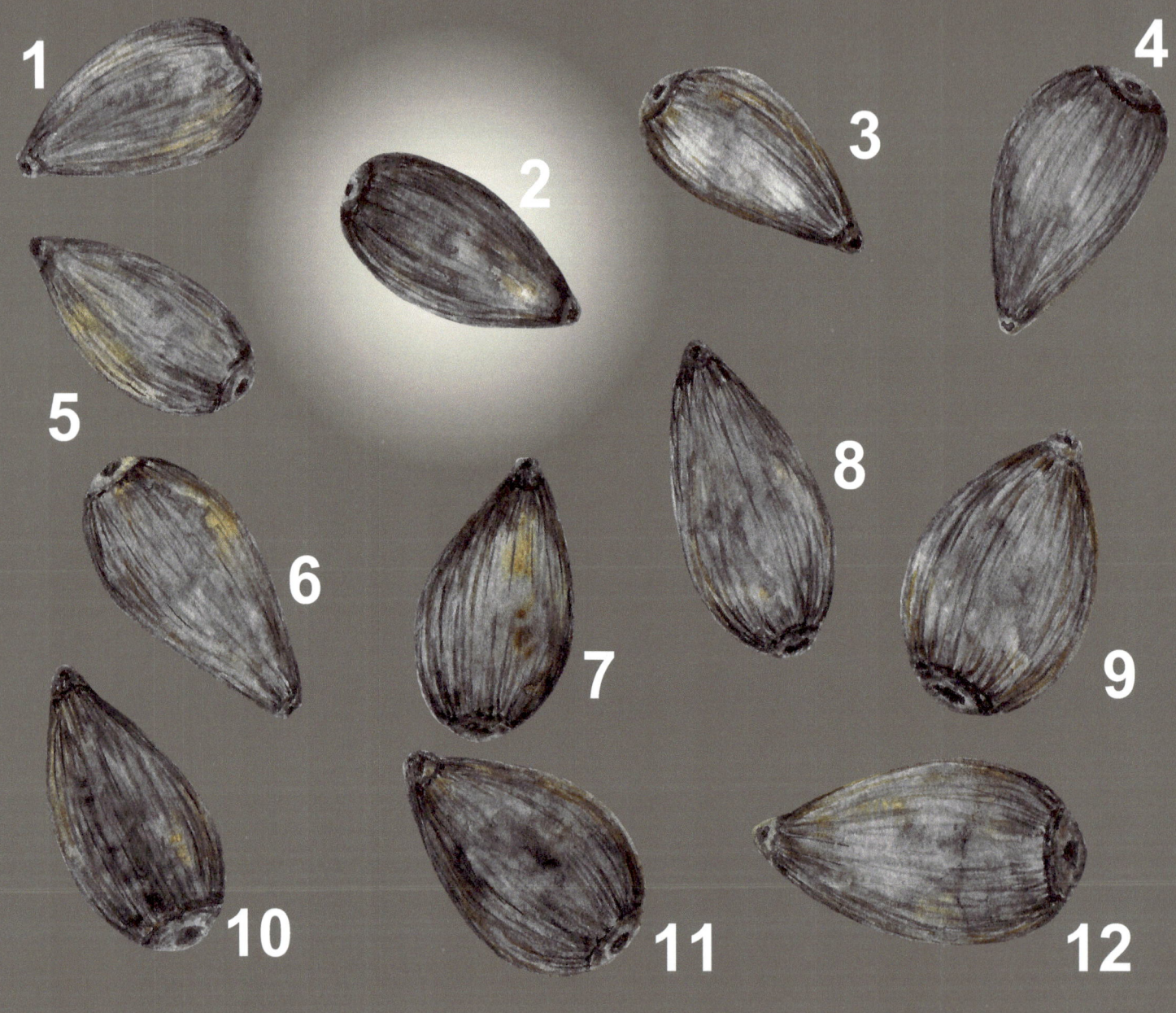

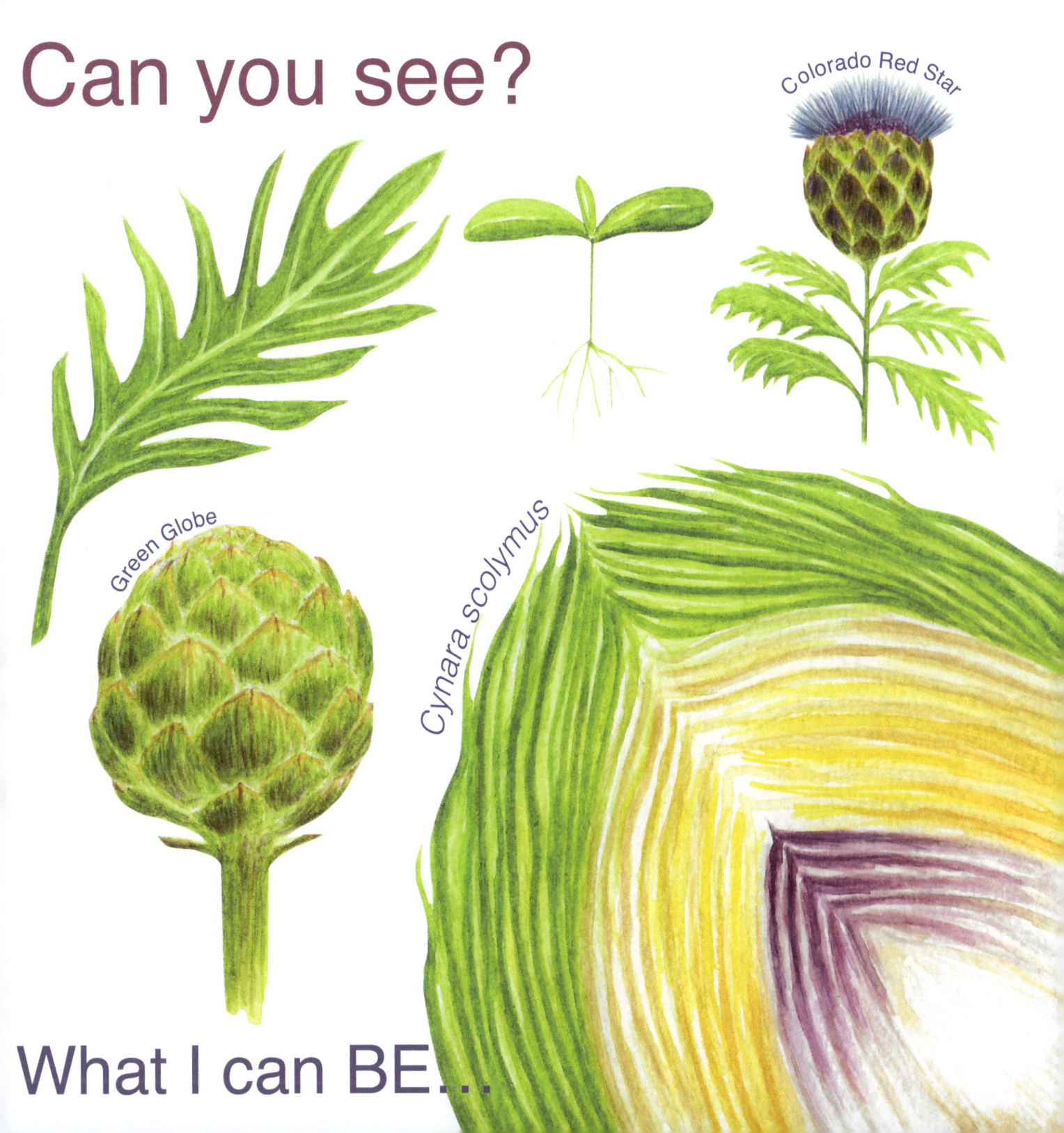

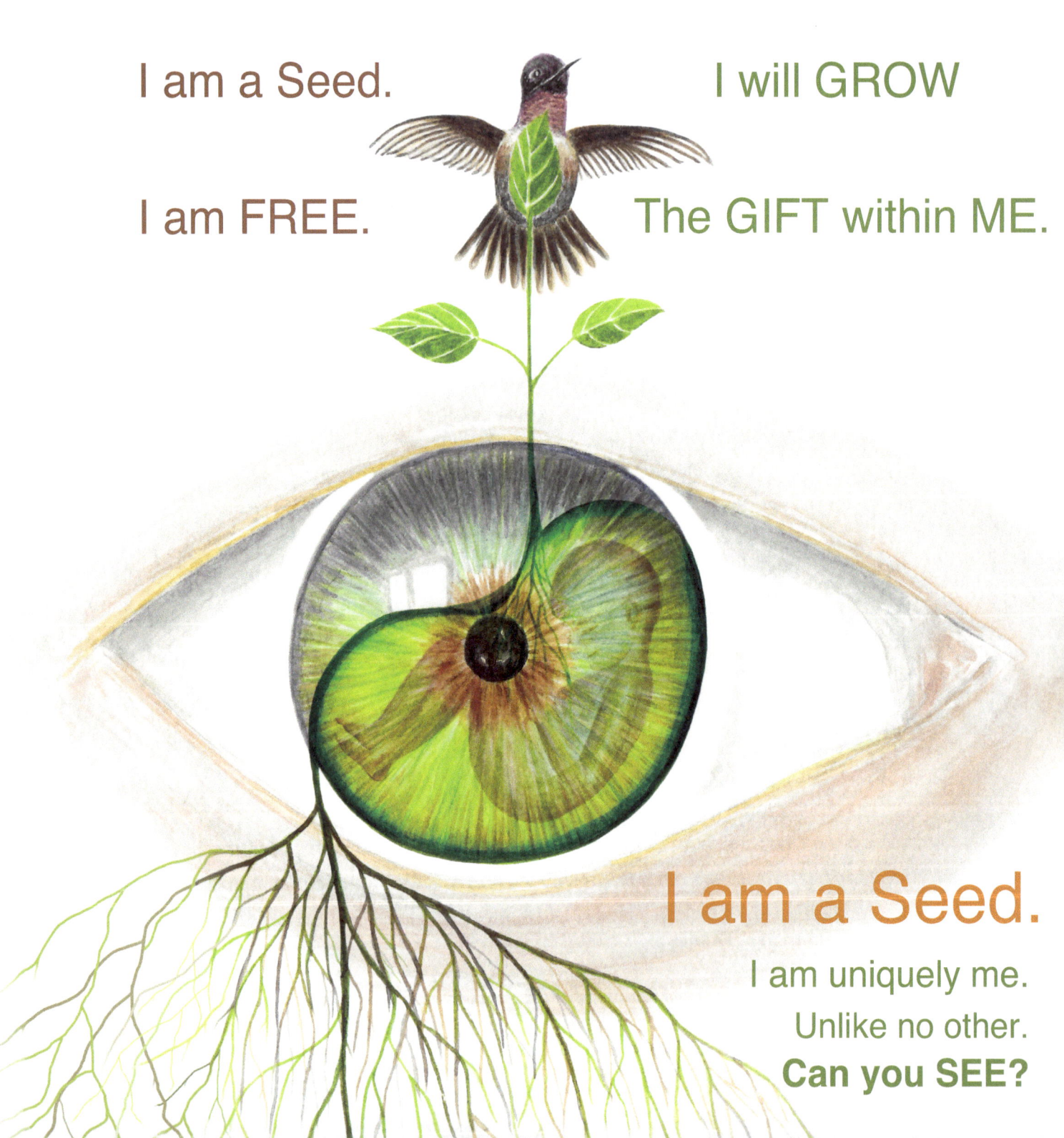

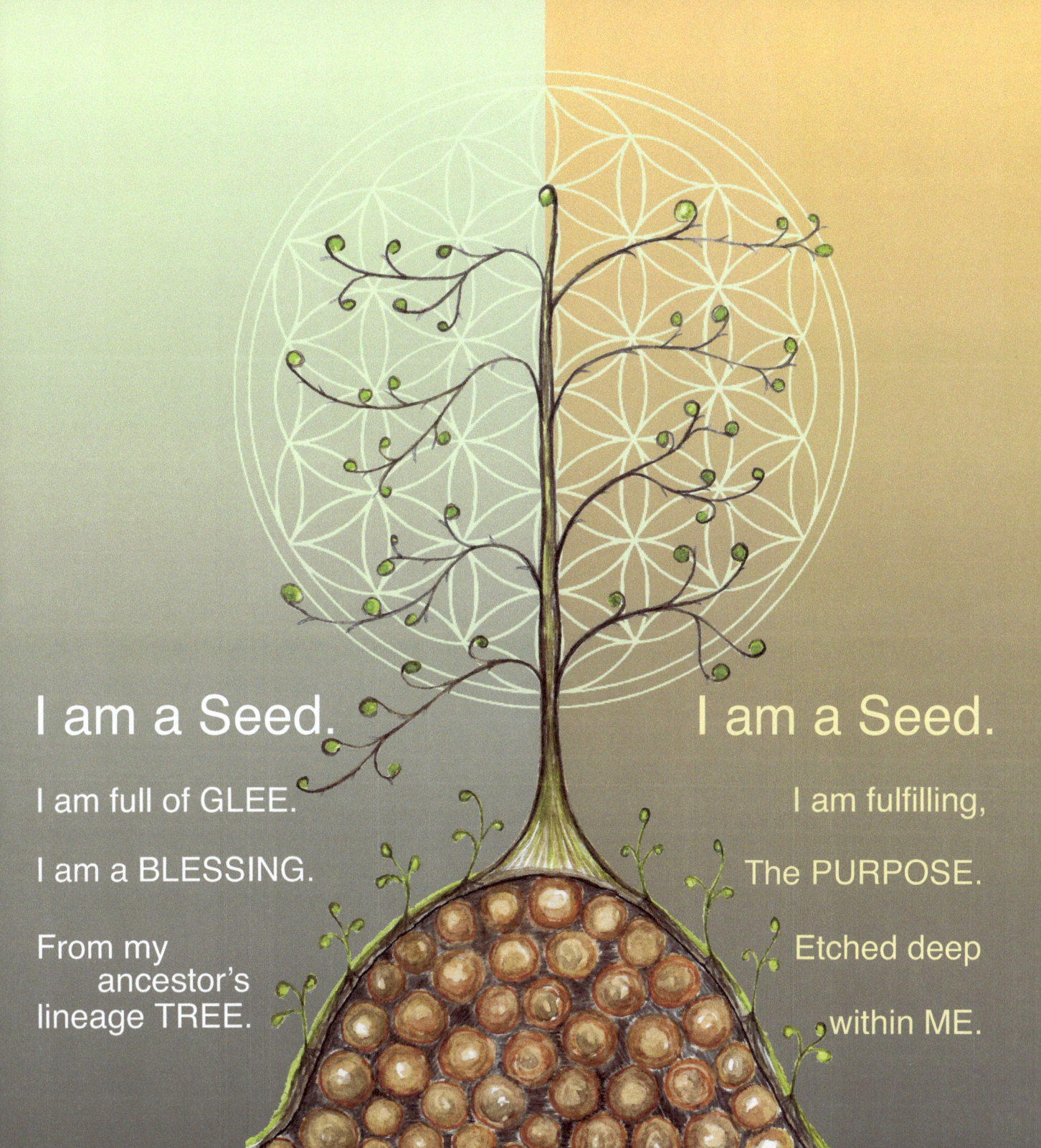

I am a Seed.

I am full of GLEE.

I am a BLESSING.

From my ancestor's lineage TREE.

I am a Seed.

I am fulfilling,

The PURPOSE.

Etched deep

within ME.

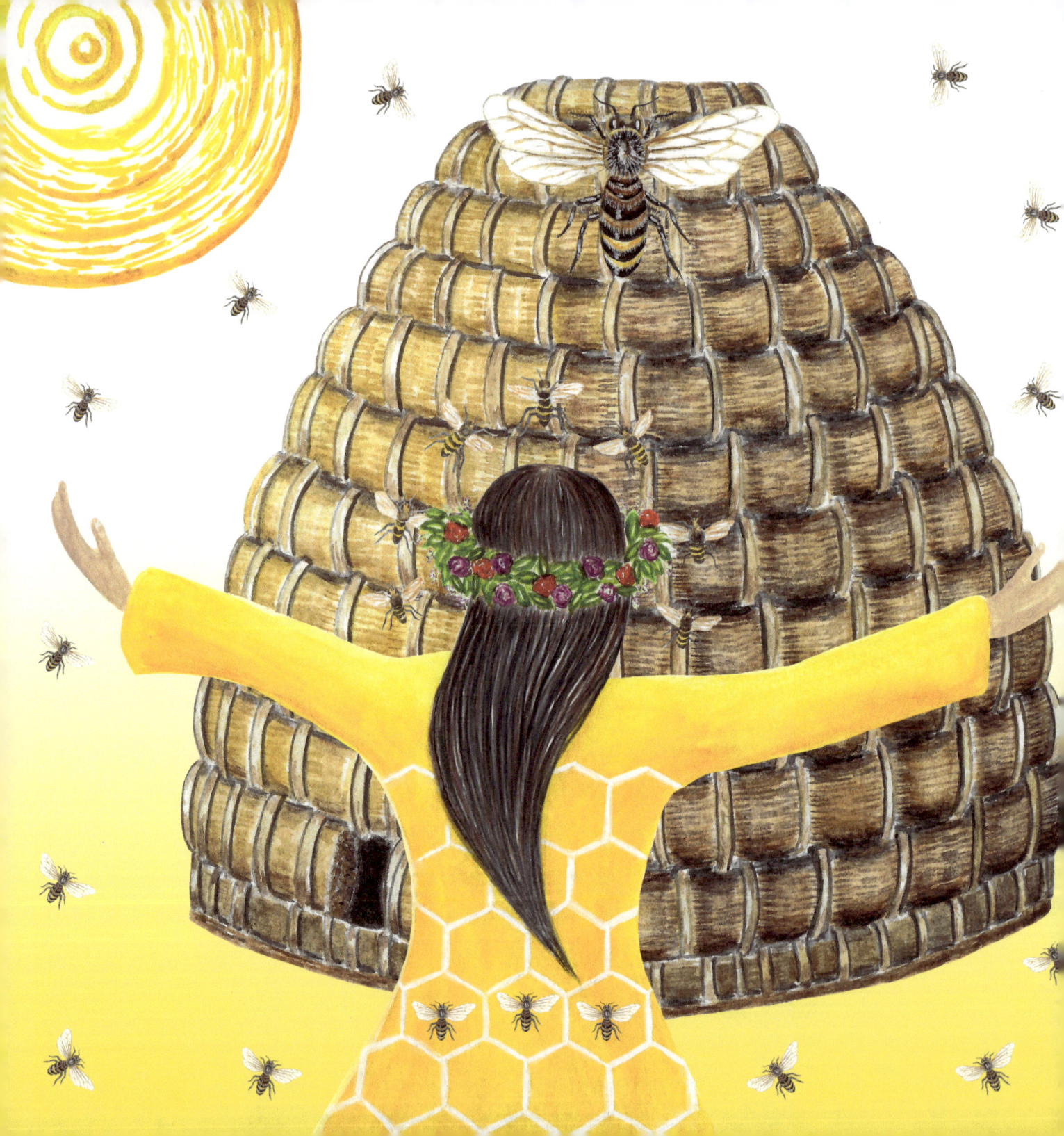

I Am a SEED.

I embrace me.

And the mission to co-create with Nature.

Just like the bee.

I Am a SEED.

And I agree.

With the power of LOVE.

That created you and me.

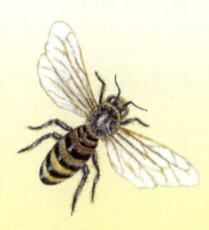
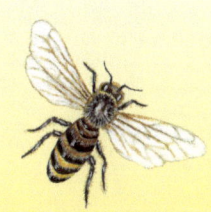
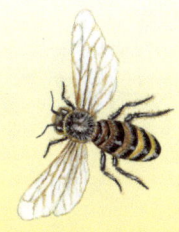
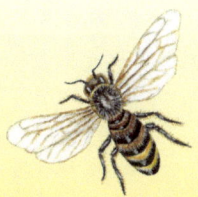
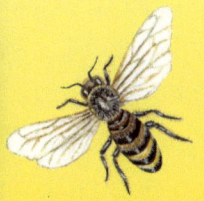
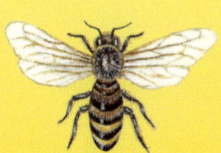
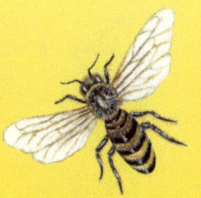
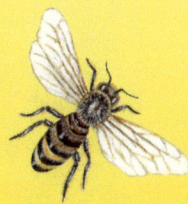

I Am a SEED.

Now you can see.

We are ONE.

Created by the same

ENERGY.

I Am a SEED.

I am COMPLETE within me.

I am one with every creature.

In HARMONY.

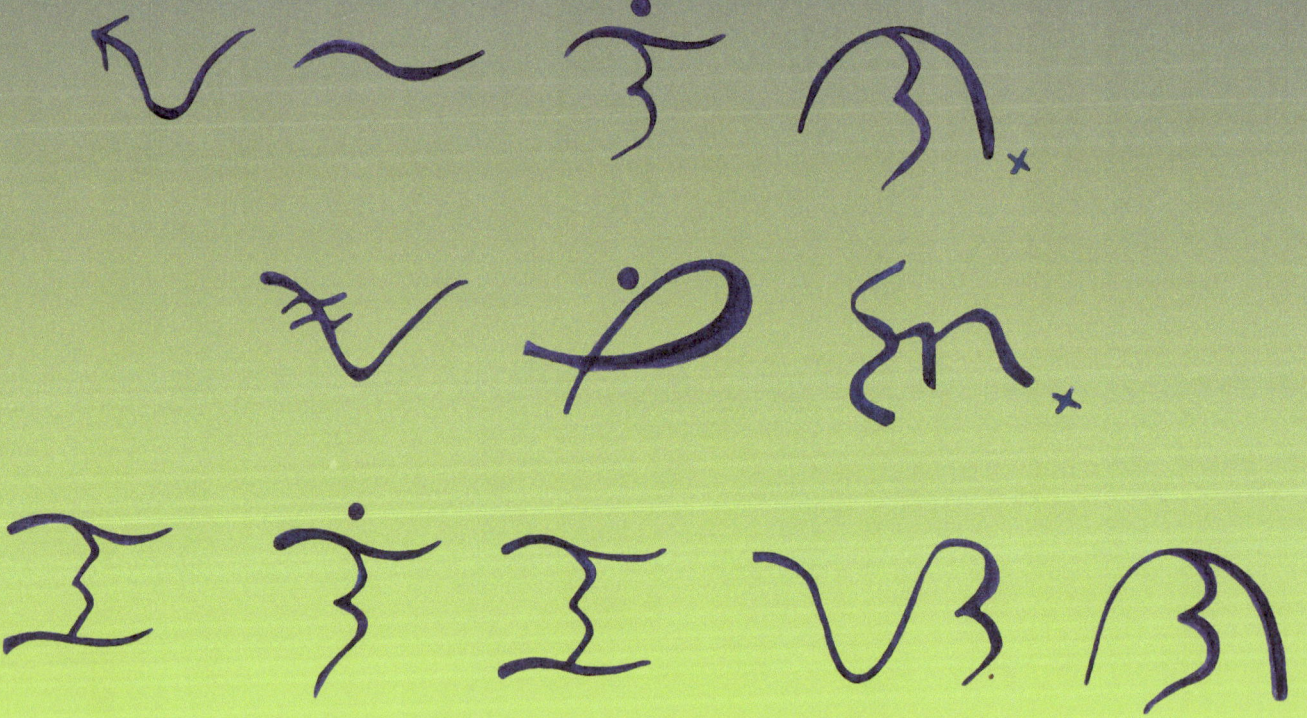

(*Baybayin:* An ancient writing system from the Philippines)

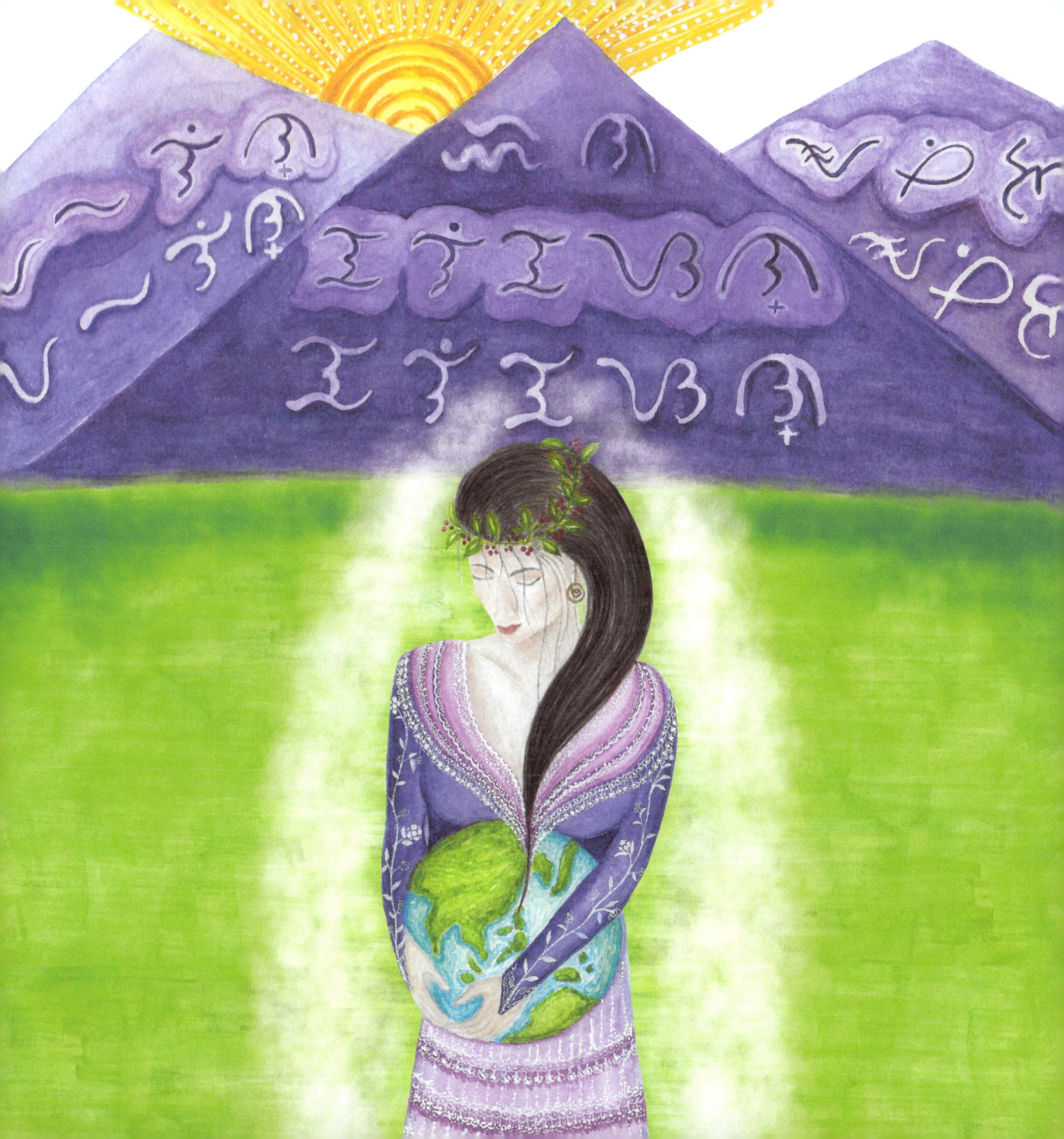

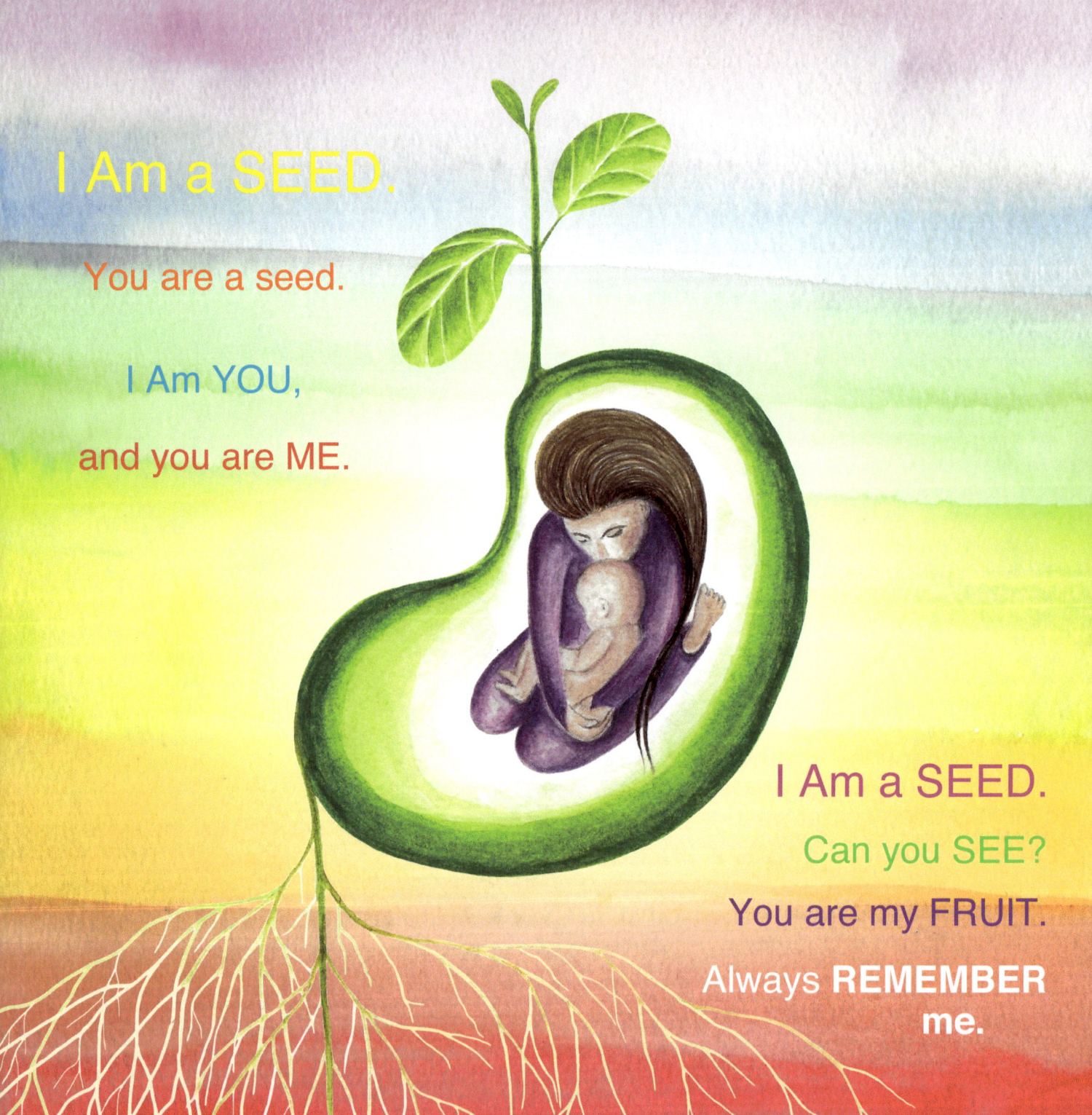

AFTERWORD
Saving our Seeds, Saving our Future
By Quin Shakra

My fascination with seeds originated during my first visits to seed farms. I thought highly of my relationship with plants at the time, but it was at those farms that I became aware of how little I knew.

There, I saw plants in forms I couldn't recognize. Plants that were reproducing; they had gone to seed. It made me realize how an entire phase of life was so unknown to me and it was during those visits that my friends and I felt sure that we were going to start a seed company.

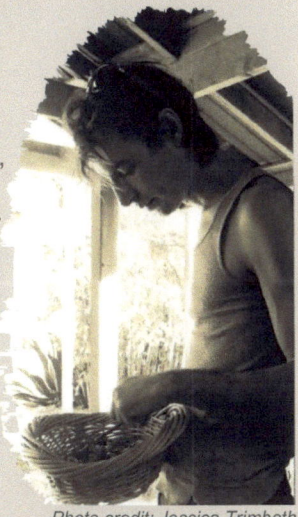

Photo credit: Jessica Trimbath

And we did, and it's still here, and I am grateful every single day that this work has found me. Plants have always been personal to me. From my early fascination with wild plant identification, to understanding the healing and edible properties of these plants, through wanting to grow every purple vegetable variety under the sun, it has always been about seeing these plants through to the point that fascinated me in the first place.

Seed saving allowed me to take that fascination to the next level. I started with what fascinated me and ended with what began the fascination.

'My simple thesis is that we save life we understand and we ignore what we don't. So please, strive to understand this life, from beginning to end....seed to seed.'

Quin Shakra is the owner and co-founder of The Plant Good Seed Company in Ojai, CA. He's been a farmer for over 17 years starting at Mano Farm in Ojai, CA since 2006. His favorite vegetable to grow from seed is squash.

About the Author

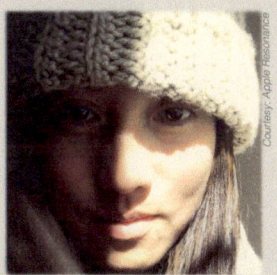

Apple (Chan) Resonance was born and raised in Manila, Philippines. She studied Interior Design at the University of the Philippines, Diliman. And was studying Masters in Interior Design when she moved to Los Angeles, CA. Not knowing she will fall in love with vegetable gardening, seed-saving and painting her vegetable harvests from her guerilla garden in Brentwood. Then from their ranch and homestead garden in Topanga. And later on, from her simple herb and vegetable garden in Big Bear, California.

Apple started saving seeds in 2009 when she met Mr. David King, founder of SLOLA (Seed Library of the Los Angeles) and all the other seed stewards at the Ojai Seed Swap. Since then, her interest in learning how to save seeds has grown immensely that led her to a spiritual journey and artistic co-creation with nature.

For this book, Apple used Sennelier watercolor, melted snow and lake water from Big Bear Lake and Lake Arrowhead.

Apple is also a conservation artist and author-illustrator of several illustrated books that promote awareness on vegetable gardening, seed-saving and eco-spirituality. She is a contributing artist for ABUN (Artists and Biologists Unite for Nature) since 2019.

Apple's favorite vegetable seeds to grow are:
Tomato, Cucumber, Carrots, Ampalaya (Bitter Melon), Spinach, Rainbow Swiss Chard, Zucchini, Beans and Bok Choy.

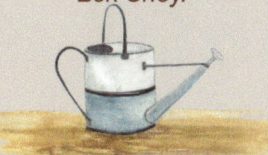

RESOURCES:

Seed companies carrying NON-GMO, heirloom and organic seeds:

Baker Creek Heirloom Seed Company
Website: https://www.rareseeds.com/
Address: 2278 Baker Creek Rd, Mansfield, MO 65704
Phone: (417) 924-8917
Email: seeds@rareseeds.com

Hardy Seeds
Website: https://growhardyseeds.com/
Address: Jackson County, Oregon
Phone: (541) 301-6447
Email: growhardyseeds@gmail.com

High Mowing Organic Seeds
Website: https://www.highmowingseeds.com/
Address: 76 Quarry Road, Wolcott, VT 05680
Phone: (866) 735-4454

The Plant Good Seed
Website: https://www.plantgoodseed.com/
Address: 226 West Ojai Ave Ste 101-539 Ojai, CA 93023
Phone: (805) 705-9550

Pinetree Seeds
Website: https://www.superseeds.com/
Address: P.O. Box 300 New Gloucester, Maine 04260
Phone: (207) 926-3400

Portland Seedhouse
Website: https://portlandseedhouse.com/
Address: Portland, Oregon
Phone: (971) 282-7181
Email: evangregoirepdx@gmail.com

Renee's Garden Seeds
Website: https://www.reneesgarden.com/
Address: 6060 Graham Hill Rd. Felton, CA 95018
Phone: 1-888-880-7228

Seed Savers Exchange Heirloom Seeds
Website: https://www.seedsavers.org/
Address: 3094 North Winn Road, Decorah, Iowa 52101
Phone: (563) 382-5990

Siskiyou Seeds
Website: https://www.siskiyouseeds.com/
Address: 3220 E Fork Rd, Williams, OR 97544
Phone: (541) 415-0877
Email: info@siskiyouseeds.com

Small House Farm
Website: https://smallhousefarm.com/
Address: 2603 W Olson Rd, Sanford, MI
Phone: (989) 708-0549
Email: SmallHouseFarm@gmail.com

Southern Exposure Seed Exchange
Website: https://www.southernexposure.com/
Address: P.O. Box 460, Mineral, Virginia 23117
Phone: (540) 894-9480

Seed Advocates and Seed Libraries:

Food is Free Project
Website: https://foodisfreeproject.org

Free Heirloom Seeds
Website: https://freeheirloomseeds.org

MI (Michigan) Seed Library Network
Website: https://miseedlibrary.org

SLOLA (Seed Library of Los Angeles)
Website: https://slola.org

The National Heirloom Exposition
Website: https://theheirloomexpo.com

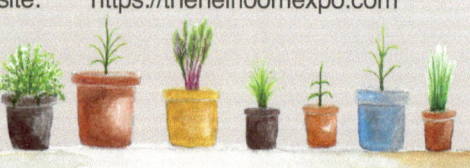

Books by Apple Resonance:

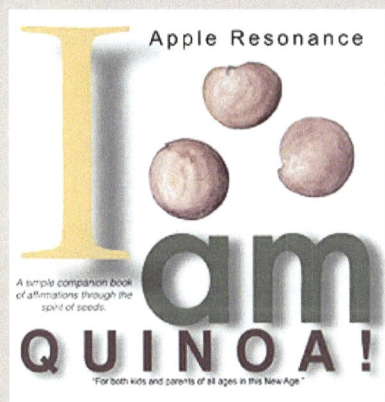
I Am Quinoa!

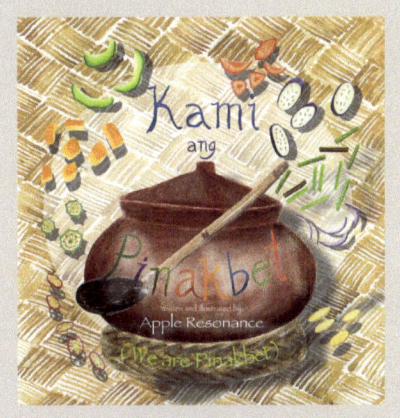
Kami Ang Pinakbet

More upcoming books by Apple Resonance:

I Am My Garden!

Every Child's Vegetable Gardening Journal

The Blue Baobab

The Street Sweeper

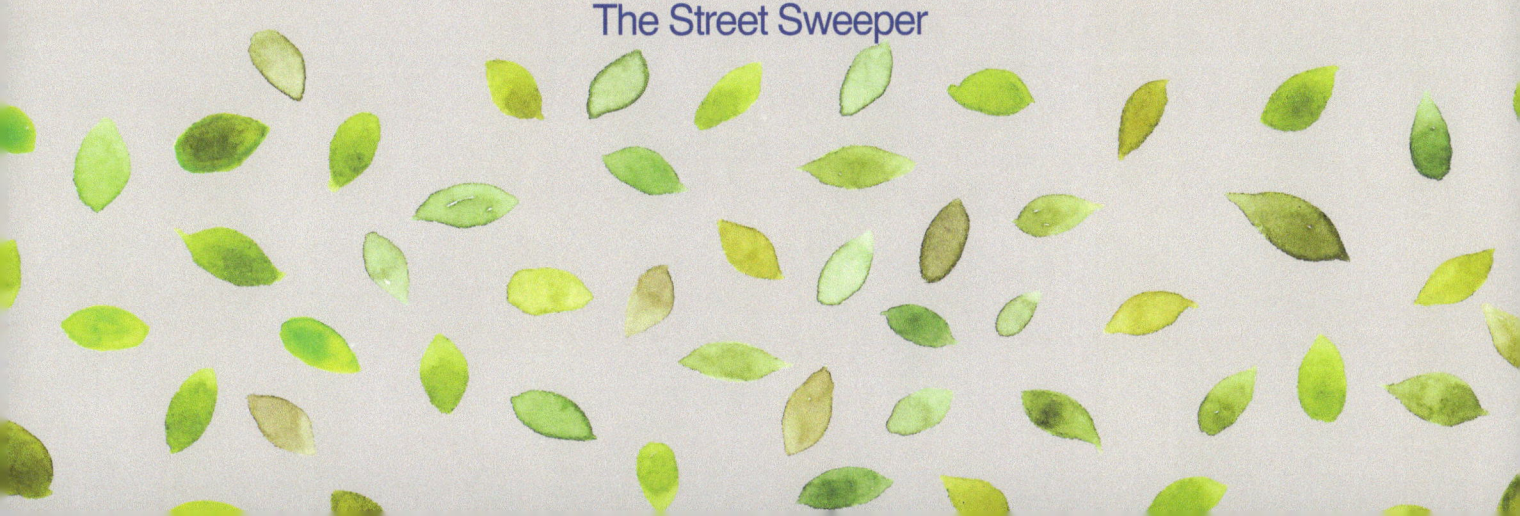

Whether you tend a garden or not,
YOU are the gardener of you own BEING.
The SEEDS of your DESTINY.

—The Findhorn Foundation

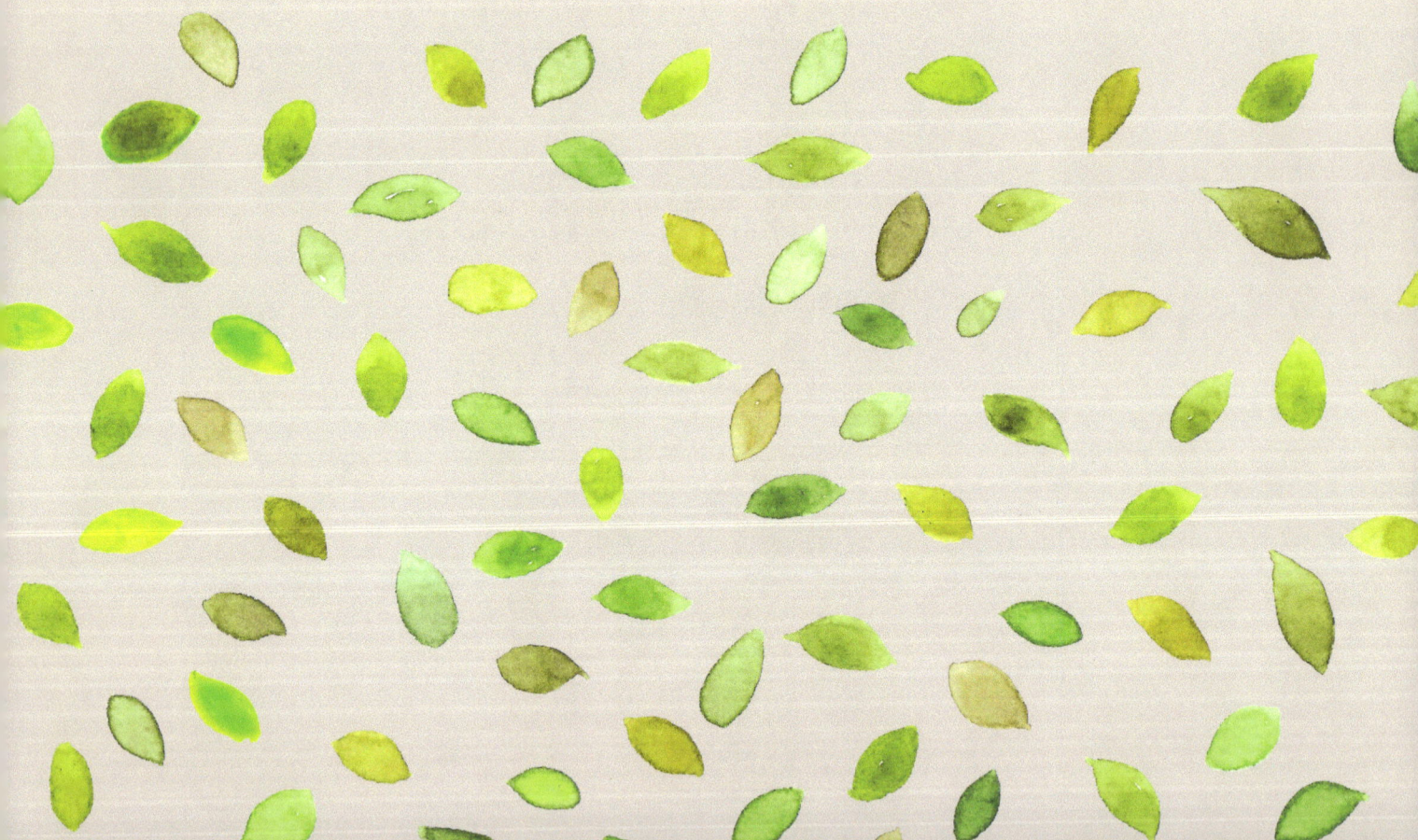

www.ingramcontent.com/pod-product-compliance
Lightning Source LLC
LaVergne TN
LVHW072114070426
835510LV00002B/55